HEART MUSCLE

ULTRASTRUCTURAL STUDIES

VISVAN NAVARATNAM

*Fellow and Director of Medical Studies, Christ's College, Cambridge
and University Lecturer in Anatomy*

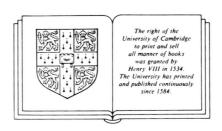

The right of the
University of Cambridge
to print and sell
all manner of books
was granted by
Henry VIII in 1534.
The University has printed
and published continuously
since 1584.

CAMBRIDGE UNIVERSITY PRESS
Cambridge
New York   New Rochelle
Melbourne   Sydney

Published by the Press Syndicate of the University of Cambridge
The Pitt Building, Trumpington Street, Cambridge CB2 1RP
32 East 57th Street, New York, NY 10022, USA
10 Stamford Road, Oakleigh, Melbourne 3166, Australia

First published 1987

Printed in Great Britain at the University Press, Cambridge

British Library cataloguing in publication data
Navaratnam, Visvan
Heart muscle: ultrastructural studies.
1. Heart – Muscle   2. Mammals –
Physiology
I. Title
599.01'16   QP113.2

Library of Congress cataloguing in publication data
Navaratnam, Visvan.
Heart muscle.

Bibliography
Includes index.
1. Heart – Muscle – Ultrastructure.   I. Title.
[DNLM: 1. Myocardium – ultrastructure.   WG 280 N319h]
QM570.5.N38 1988   599'.0116   87–13205

ISBN 0 521 24965 1

WV

CONTENTS

PREFACE

Although the strength and rate of cardiac contractions are capable
of variation over a substantial range, such fluctuations usually are
temporary episodes and the heart normally reverts to a steady level
of performance. The underlying consistency of the heart beat has
intrigued generations of scientific observers from ancient times and
the Edwin Smith Surgical Papyrus records that it attracted comment
as early as 3000–2500 B.C. Among others, Aristotle (384–322
B.C.) perceived the vital role of the heart and commented that it was
the first organ to live and the last to die. Galileo (1564–1642) was so
impressed with the regularity of the pulse that he used it to check the
consistency of pendulum swing.

We now know that, despite the manifest reliability of myocardial
action as a whole, its constituent cells exhibit considerable variability of performance. The concept that heart muscle is composed of
separate cells did not become firmly established till after the advent
of the electron microscope in the middle of the present century. The
co-ordination of myriad myocytes, varying in excitability and
conductivity as well as in contractility, is a remarkable exercise in
harmony. Phylogenetically, the earliest effective hearts are to be
found among annelid worms and, in almost all species endowed
with a heart, the generation and conduction of the cardiac impulse
have been shown to be intrinsic to the musculature. In such
myogenic hearts there usually exists a hierarchy of cells varying in
spontaneous excitability, the variation being dependent on differences in ionic permeability of the sarcolemma. The most excit-

able myocytes depolarise to generate the cardiac impulse and they recruit their less-excitable neighbours before the latter are spontaneously able to depolarise. Cell-to-cell transmission is effected by functional coupling which is held to be dependent on specialised membrane junctions such as nexuses (gap junctions). Investigations of sarcolemmal permeability, cell-to-cell conduction and excitation-contraction coupling in cardiac myocytes have been foci of intense activity over the past decade.

Such advances emphasise that detailed knowledge of the fine structure of cardiac myocytes, their subcellular components and intercellular contacts is highly desirable for an understanding of the co-ordinated performance of the heart. The material presented in the succeeding chapters of this monograph comprises investigations conducted in the author's laboratory on ultrastructural features of mammalian heart muscle which bear on its functional performance. A number of features are included but the coverage is by no means complete; for instance, little emphasis is afforded to nuclei of cardiac myocytes or to extracellular ground substance while most attention is directed to cytoplasmic organelles and to the sarcolemma. The initial chapter is devoted to differentiation of the embryonic myocardial rudiment in the mouse which is probably the most convenient material for the study of mammalian organogenesis. Next, the ultrastructure of typical definitive myocardial cells is considered in Chapter 2 and followed by four chapters on specialised features, namely nexuses, T-tubules, storage organelles and atrial specific granules. Most of the descriptions are of material from small mammals such as the mouse, rat and hamster, and prepared in the laboratory. Some human material obtained by biopsy during surgery has also been studied but the interests of the patient do not permit removal or fixation in a manner optimal for ultrastructural study.

The central mechanical role played by the heart in pumping blood to other organs entails problems for its own metabolic requirements for, while there is metabolic demand anywhere in the body, the heart is required to continue its action even during hypoxic conditions such as those imposed by severe physical exercise. Heart muscle is able to cope with such demands by means of features including cellular metabolic adaptations and enhanced coronary vascularisation. Enormous impetus for the study of myocardial metabolism has been provided by modern advances in surgical technique wherein the heart may be put through procedures such as perfusion, cardioplegic arrest and hypothermia in preparation for by-pass surgery or for transplantation. The emergence of non-invasive techniques such as nuclear magnetic resonance spectroscopy in the study of tissue metabolism has sustained the boost in interest and has provided further incentives. The effects of ischaemic arrest with or without perfusion and hypothermia are discussed in Chapter 5, following consideration of storage organelles.

In recent years it has become clear that the heart does play wide-ranging roles in the maintenance of homeostasis and Chapter 6 is addressed to this issue. Some cardiac myocytes, especially those in the auricular appendages of several mammalian species, are characterised by the presence of peptide-containing granules in the cytoplasm. There is evidence that these cells, in response to volume distension of the circulation, release a specific principle (atriopeptin) which promotes the excretion of salt and water from the body thus relieving the circulatory load. It has also been demonstrated that a peptide of the same chemical structure is found in neurons within several regions of the brain and, interestingly enough, many of these regions are known or suspected to be concerned with cardiovascular regulation or with fluid and electrolyte balance.

Chapter 7 is devoted to ageing changes in cardiac myocytes and Chapter 8 to the ultrastructural features of myocardial innervation. The remarkable basic regularity of the heart, in regard to rate and strength of contraction, is dependent to a substantial extent on physiological responses to oscillations of those parameters. The heart may be myogenically driven but it is modulated by neuronal reflexes triggered by the ability to sense changes in pressure on the venous and arterial sides of the circulation. In response, the nervous system exerts restitutions in the contractile performance of the myocardium. Such feedback mechanisms modulating the haemodynamic performance of the heart are crucial for the homeostasis of the organism. Moreover, the nervous system has the capacity to alter cardiac performance within limits in response to physiological demands. Over the past decade or so, knowledge of visceral innervation including that of the heart has expanded substantially, especially with the advent of suitable immunochemical techniques, and any discussion on heart muscle necessitates an up-to-date review of cardiac innervation, cardiac neurotransmitters and the relevant receptors. An attempt has been made to summarise this information in the final chapter of this volume. Heart muscle is also directly affected by circulating substances such as catecholamines and thyroid hormones; these substances may affect not only the short term contractile performance of cardiac myocytes, thus supplementing neuronal mechanisms, but also their long term differentiation and growth.

The literature on myocardial ultrastructure is very extensive and hence the bibliography in this book is likely to fall short of doing justice to all worthy contributions. Where satisfactory reviews are available, the reader will be referred to these and provided with recent supplementary references. For instance, in Chapter 2 much of the literature before 1979 has been omitted because it has been reviewed in excellent and comprehensive publications by Challice & Virágh (1973) and by Sommer & Johnson (1979). A recent book *Cardiac Muscle* by Canale, Campbell, Smolich & Campbell (1986) considers how cultured cardiac myocytes may be used as models for research.

The scope of the present publication does not permit detailed accounts of the methodology of ultrastructural or cytochemical techniques but appropriate features of technique will be discussed where the interpretation of appearance is at issue. Wherever possible, readers will be referred to source articles which should be consulted for details.

Christ's College   V. Navaratnam
Cambridge   *January 1987*

ACKNOWLEDGEMENTS

This book would not have been possible without the collaboration and encouragement of Jeremy Skepper, Ken Thurley, Seth Ayettey, Matt Kaufman, Martin Feldman, Daniel Hill, Keith Guttridge, Tim Crane, Susan Insole, Anne Wright and of many other colleagues too numerous to be listed here. I am much indebted to the British Heart Foundation for their generous support of the work from its early stages and especially for donating the freeze-fracture apparatus. I am also grateful to the managers of the Charles Slater Fund for a grant to cover secretarial assistance and the literature search and to Dr Ayris of the Scientific Periodicals Library in Cambridge for executing the search. Most of all, I must thank my wife Sundari and my daughters for putting up with so many demands, many of them quite unreasonable, during preparation of the text.

1

Differentiation of the myocardial rudiment in mouse embryos

Many of the original workers in the field of vertebrate cardiac development studied the embryology of the mammalian heart (e.g. human: Davis, 1927; rat: Goss, 1938, 1952; guinea-pig: Yoshinaga, 1921; rabbit: Van der Stricht, 1895) and it was shown that the first cardiac contractions occur during the early somite stage of development just as the previously bilateral endocardial tubes coalesce in the midline. Other investigators, however, examined chick and duck hearts to provide a descriptive account of early cardiac morphogenesis (duck: Yoshida, 1932; chick: Sabin, 1920; Patten & Kramer, 1933; De Haan, 1964, 1965; Argüello, de la Cruz & Gómez, 1975; Manasek, 1976). Indeed much of the recent work on cardiac morphogenesis has concentrated on the ultrastructure of the avian heart probably because of its convenience of access. However, fundamental differences exist between cardiogenesis in birds and in mammals particularly in the timing of the first appearance of the pericardial cavity. In the avian embryo two amniocardiac vesicles initially appear at about the 1- to 3-somite stage, and median fusion occurs at about the 9-somite stage; likewise, in the avian embryo, the primitive cardiac cells are thought to migrate to the presumptive pericardial cavity (De Haan, 1964, 1965; Rosenquist & De Haan, 1966). In mammals, the presumptive pericardial cavity appears at a considerably earlier stage of embryogenesis, and the primitive cardiac rudiments are thought to differentiate *in situ* (see Yoshinaga, 1921; Davis, 1927).

Although small laboratory mammals such as the mouse have

become increasingly convenient and valuable for embryological research, there are relatively few ultrastructural accounts in the literature with information on the intra- and extra-cellular changes that occur during differentiation of the early myocardial rudiment in mammals. Attempts to close this gap in knowledge have been made in articles on mouse embryos by Challice & Virágh (1973) and by Navaratnam, Kaufman, Skepper, Barton & Guttridge (1986). This chapter comprises a detailed description of the differentiation of myocardial elements and their precursor anlage in mouse embryos from the eighth day of gestation (i.e. before cardiac contractions have commenced and indeed even before a myocardial rudiment can be recognised), through later stages of embryonic development to the first day of the postnatal period. Detailed attention is paid to the 8–9-day period. Among other matters, the account confirms that the myocardial plate differentiates *in situ* as a thickening of part of the splanchnic pericardial lining at the presomite stage of development, on the afternoon or evening of the eighth day of pregnancy. Since gap junctions (nexuses) are widely believed to be the basis of cell-to-cell conduction of the cardiac impulse, close attention has been paid to the sequence in which such cell junctions are assembled in the myocardial plate both before and during the stages of development when the earliest contractions are established. The description is principally based on transmission electron microscopy of ultrathin sections but it is supplemented, for some suitable embryonic stages of development, by light microscopy of semithin plastic sections as well as scanning electron microscopy (Kaufman & Navaratnam, 1981) and analysis of freeze-fracture replicas (Navaratnam, Skepper & Thurley, 1980).

Although no absolute correlation exists between the degree of development of the heart and the number of somites, for descriptive purposes it has proved convenient to group the early embryos according to the state of somite morphogenesis. It should be emphasised, nevertheless, that some degree of overlap in regard to cardiac differentiation is observed when such a classification is employed (Kaufman & Navaratnam, 1981).

Presomite headfold stages

In embryos isolated on the afternoon or early evening of the eighth day of pregnancy, examination of semithin plastic sections reveals one or more narrow spaces (Fig. 1.1) in the mesoderm between the most proximal part of the headfolds and the attachment of the amnion in this region. Initially these spaces, which comprise the earliest anlage of the pericardial coelom, are lined by flattened mesothelial cells abutting against each other without much overlap.

In some embryos of this group, typically those isolated late on the evening of the eighth day of pregnancy (i.e. corresponding to late headfold stage), there is a recognisable thickening of the lining on the ventral aspect of the pericardium where the cells had become plump, though still forming a single layer; this thickened area comprises the rudimentary myocardial epithelium or plate.

The surface plasmalemma of these cells is covered by a flocculent basement membrane which is thickest at the basal or abluminal aspect of each cell. Otherwise the basal surfaces are relatively featureless and they comprise an undulant border with few processes. On the other hand, the apical surface which lines the presumptive pericardial sac invariably possesses short, irregularly spaced microvilli (Fig. 1.2) some of which terminate in bulbous heads. The lateral surfaces, where adjacent cells appose each other, are relatively short at this stage of development in keeping with the flattened nature of the cells. Apposition is closest near the pericardial lumen (Figs. 1.2, 1.3) where specialised junctional features can be discerned. These contacts resemble desmosomes in that the apposing membranes are flanked by cytoplasmic strips of enhanced density but, unlike typical definitive desmosomes, no intercellular density is identifiable as yet; nor is there evidence of cytoplasmic filaments inserted into the membranes at these sites. Near such desmosome-like junctions, but further away from the pericardial lumen, there are punctate sites where the gap between adjacent cell membranes is reduced to much less than 20 nm and occasionally there are spots where the gap seems to be obliterated and cannot be visualised even after tilting of the specimen in the electron microscope.

The cytoplasmic matrix of these cells is studded with electron-dense ribosomal granules, possessing an angular profile and measuring 12–18 nm across (Figs. 1.3, 1.4). Some are distributed singly but most are grouped to form typical rosette-like polysomes. In addition, there are larger (30 nm in diameter), more rounded granules which are probably glycogen granules; these are not frequently found in aggregation. A few mitochondria are dispersed in the cytoplasm which also contains some spherical droplets of various sizes (Fig. 1.3). Most of the content of each droplet is electron-lucent but there is some dense material at the centre of the smaller droplets. The smaller, presumably immature, droplets are situated near the extremities of the Golgi apparatus indicating their probable origin from the latter, whilst the larger droplets have

Fig. 1.1. Transverse section through the upper headfold region of a late presomite mouse embryo isolated on the afternoon of the eighth day of gestation. Narrow spaces (P) lined by flattened cells are present in the mesoderm of the presumptive pericardial region. These represent the rudiments of the pericardial cavity which later coalesce to form a single cavity. Photograph by courtesy of Professor M.H. Kaufman.

Fig. 1.2. Transmission electron micrograph showing cells lining the ventral aspect of the pericardial cavity (P). Note the short microvilli on the pericardial aspect of these cells and the apposition of their lateral walls, including a junctional complex (arrow) near the pericardial lumen.

Fig. 1.3. Evening of the eighth day. The cells lining the ventral aspect of the pericardial sac (P) have become elongated and their cytoplasm is studded with numerous granules including monosomes and polysomes. The picture also shows several other granules and droplets, starting near the Golgi apparatus with mainly electron-dense material while the larger droplets, containing predominantly electron-lucent material, have migrated to the periphery. They are surrounded by a halo of ribosomes.

Fig. 1.4. Eighth day evening, presomite mouse embryo. Cytoplasm of an elongated cell on the ventral wall of the pericardium. Apart from numerous ribosomes in the cytoplasm there are fine filaments which are occasionally found in small fascicles (F).

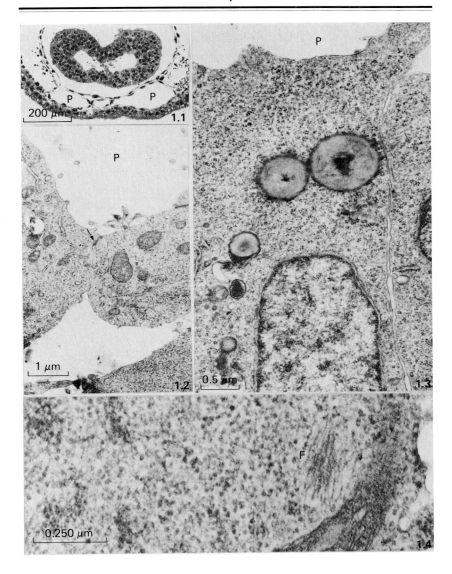

moved away towards the periphery of the cells; the limiting membranes of the larger droplets have become attenuated and indistinct and there is a surrounding halo of densely aggregated ribosomes. Large droplets are found most often near the pericardial aspect of the cells but, not infrequently, they are found near the basal and lateral surfaces as well. Some are found very close to the cell membrane. The endoplasmic reticulum (ER) is not particularly prominent at this stage; there are a few elongated and apparently unorientated cisterns (Fig. 1.2), mostly of the granular variety with ribosomes inserted on their membranes. The occasional cistern is situated close to the cell surface, especially near the lateral borders between apposed cells, but there is no clear evidence of intraluminal or cytoplasmic densities which characterise definitive couplings between sarcoplasmic reticulum and sarcolemma (Ayettey & Navaratnam, 1978). Nor are there any invaginations of the surface membrane such as T-tubules or caveolae. However, there are several coated vesicles, some of which are attached to the cell surface while others are pinched off into the cytoplasm.

In addition to the granules and larger organelles, the cytoplasm also contains some fine filamentous material. Most of the latter is dispersed irregularly but, occasionally, short fascicles of parallel filaments measuring 6–7 nm in thickness can be identified (Fig. 1.4) especially near the lateral borders of the cell. Fascicles of this type are more easily identified in association with the spindle apparatus in cells undergoing mitosis but they are also present in resting cells.

Owing to the minute size of the presumptive pericardial coelom at the presomite stage of development, it was not possible to locate the lining cells or the rudimentary myocardial plate in freeze-fracture preparations of embryos in this group; nor was it possible for technical reasons to locate the coelomic/pericardial rudiments in scanning preparations.

Embryos with 1–2 pairs of somites

This group comprises embryos isolated early on the morning of the ninth day of gestation, by which time the pericardial sac has widened and is continuous across the midline extending on either side of the foregut pocket. The ventral lining of the sac is thickened to form the myocardial plate in all specimens (Fig. 1.5) and, in some embryos, the plate is raised on either side of the midline forming a pair of approximately symmetrical elevations. The thickened plate initially comprises a single layer of cuboidal or columnar cells many of which show mitotic activity. In some embryos more than a single layer of cells can be discerned in parts of the plate. Immediately subjacent to the myocardial plate, there are separate cells which can be identified as presumptive endocardial elements. These cells are more flattened and elongated than the myocardial elements and are often found to be grouped round small spaces which subsequently coalesce in a predominantly antero-ventral direction round the developing foregut pocket. In certain specimens cardiogenesis seems to be slightly more advanced in that the endocardial spaces have aggregated to form a pair of tubes, one on each side of the midline, that approximate to each other anterior to the foregut pocket but have not yet fused. The myocardial plate immediately overlying each endocardial tube is slightly raised into the pericardial coelom giving the appearance of the previously noted paired elevations.

Scanning electron micrographs (Fig. 1.6) show the frontal view of an early nine-day embryo in which the headfolds and foregut are clearly seen. By removing the surface ectoderm and adherent parietal pericardial components of the anterior trunk wall, it was possible to identify the relatively wide pericardial cavity and to view the ventral splanchnic wall from within. A small collection of presumptive myocardial cells is identified protruding from this wall.

At the ultrastructural level the cells of the myocardial plate appear elongated, resembling columnar epithelial cells, and they present irregularly distributed microvilli at the apical (pericardial) surface. Their lateral surfaces are remarkably straight and the intercellular spaces between individual cells are maintained at approximately 20 nm for most of their extent (Fig. 1.7). However, there are punctate sites where the space is markedly reduced. Most of these sites are nexuses because, on tilting the specimen, a gap of at least 2 nm can be resolved; they are usually limited to single points but, in some instances, there is a series of such punctate junctions interspersed with areas of looser contact (Fig. 1.8). Nevertheless, material labelled with ruthenium red (see Luft, 1971, for details of technique) revealed that there also are some tight junctions near the apices of the cells for the label is restricted to the pericardial surface of each cell and to a very short apical segment of the intercellular space (Fig. 1.9). In addition, several junctions resembling desmosomes or maculae adherentes are recognised along the lateral cell margins (Fig. 1.7). At such junctions, the intercellular space is maintained at about 20 nm and a dense line can be recognised within the space in some of them. There is increased cytoplasmic density flanking each membrane and, in some instances, filaments are found attached to the membranes at such sites. Like the nexuses and tight junctions, developing desmosomes are found most

Fig. 1.5. Transverse section through a 1–2-somite stage embryo, isolated early on the morning of the ninth day of gestation. The pericardial cavity (P) extends laterally on either side of the foregut pocket (G) and its ventral lining is thickened to form the presumptive myocardial plate (M).

Fig. 1.6. Scanning electron micrographs showing the pericardial cavity of a 1–2-somite stage embryo. A small collection of presumptive myocardial cells (arrowed) can be identified protruding from the ventral splanchnic wall of the sac. Photograph by courtesy of Professor M.H. Kaufman.

Fig. 1.7. Thin section showing apposing cells in the myocardial plate of a 1–2-somite stage embryo with junctional complexes near the pericardial lumen (P). In addition, the membranes show close apposition at occasional punctate sites (arrow). Note the numerous polysomes in the cytoplasm and the cisterns of granular endoplasmic reticulum.

Fig. 1.8. Electron micrograph showing a series of punctate nexuses (arrows) between the membranes of two apposing cells.

Fig. 1.9. Electron micrograph of material stained with ruthenium red showing apposing cells in the myocardial plate. The label is seen on the pericardial aspect (P) of the cells but it is impeded by a junctional complex from passing further down into the intercellular space.

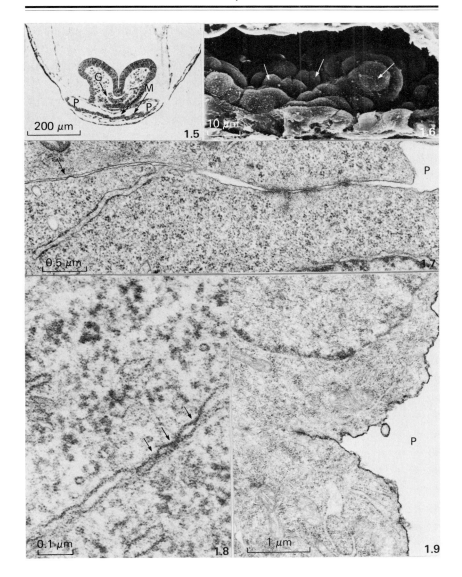

frequently near the pericardial end of each intercellular cleft but there are others, less distinct, in deeper positions.

The basement membrane or laminar coat is recognisable as an irregular flocculent layer on all aspects of the cell surface. It is thickest at the basal surface (30–120 nm) but thinnest at the pericardial surface (less than 30 nm) where in many places it is so fine that it is not easy to discern. Nowhere does the laminar coat exhibit the characteristic layered appearance which it possesses in adult cardiac myocytes (see Sommer & Johnson, 1979).

In the cytoplasm, the most conspicuous feature is the presence of numerous granules throughout (Figs. 1.7, 1.8). The preponderant variety are ribosomes, most of which are clustered in rosette form, but there are also larger glycogen-type granules which are somewhat smoother in outline. The density of granule distribution is greater than at the previous stage indicating increased synthetic activity. Numerous fine microfilaments and microtubules are scattered in the cytoplasm and, in addition, there are fascicles of longer filaments especially near the lateral cell borders. Some filaments are inserted into the cell membrane near, but not at, desmosomes indicating the formation of fasciae adherentes. There is no evidence of striation along the length of these fascicles nor of any dense patches resembling Z-lines associated with them at this stage of development.

The amount of ER present in the cytoplasm has increased in comparison to the presomite stage and most of it is of the granular variety although there are a few small smooth cisterns near the surface membrane (sarcolemma). These sub-sarcolemmal elements still lack the structural features of couplings, nor are there any caveolae or other invaginations of the sarcolemma. Mitochondria have increased in number and, in addition, there are droplets similar to those seen at the presomite stage. The latter are mostly of the large variety filled with electron-lucent material and possessing an indistinct limiting membrane surrounded by numerous polysomes. Although several small vesicles are found in association with the Golgi apparatus, their contents are clear and do not resemble the immature droplets seen at the earlier stage.

The nucleus is large and elongated like the cell itself and its nucleolus is strikingly prominent in many instances. Some of the cells contain a single cilium with constituent microtubules and basal body complex embedded in the cytoplasm. Such cilia are never encountered in mitotic cells of which there are many in the myocardial epithelium.

Freeze-fracture appearance

Localisation of the myocardial plate in freeze-fracture preparations depends to some extent on the accuracy of the initial dissection of the embryo but, in addition, the epithelium-like appearance of the myocardial plate and characteristic microvilli at its pericardial face are invaluable in its identification.

In some replicas it is possible to observe tangential views of sarcolemma and it was readily confirmed that there are no surface invaginations at this stage of development. Intramembranous particles measuring 12–14 nm in diameter are present on all surfaces and, in addition, smaller nexus (8–10 nm) particles can be recognised where the lateral surface has been exposed (Fig. 1.10). In preparations where the fracture plane has revealed the P-face and E-face of apposed membranes, it is possible to confirm that they bridge one membrane to the other (Fig. 1.11). The freeze-fracture replicas also reveal the presence of tight junctions, especially near the apical end of the lateral cell surface (Fig. 1.12). The tight junctions encountered comprise interconnected ridges and reciprocal grooves though, in some places, there is discontinuity of the constituent lines giving an appearance intermediate between those of tight junctions and nexuses. In any case there is a tendency for early nexuses to lie close to or even among the ridges and grooves of tight junctions suggesting similar sites of origin.

Embryos with 3–4 pairs of somites

Most embryos have reached the 3–4-somite stage by mid-morning on the ninth day of gestation and this is the earliest stage at which twitching of the cardiac rudiments is observed. On initial isolation of the embryos into phosphate-buffered saline, contractions are not seen but, when they are transferred to rat serum at 37°C and allowed to recover for a few minutes, irregular localised and feeble twitches can be discerned in some specimens.

The scanning electron micrographs reveal considerably enlarged myocardial thickenings which appear to be attached to the floor of the pericardial cavity (Fig. 1.14) and the caudal part of its dorsal wall. The thickenings are bilateral and the two rudiments, while in cellular continuity, are delineated by a prominent fissure in the midline.

Study of semithin plastic sections confirms that the cardiac rudiment is attached to the floor of the pericardial sac (Fig. 1.13). The rudimentary endocardial tubes consist of a single layer of flattened cells surrounding loculi of various sizes, some of which have fused together. The tubes are almost completely ensheathed by a common sleeve of myocardial tissue and between the myocardial sleeve and endocardial tubes there has now appeared a wide space

Fig. 1.10. Ninth day morning, 1–2-somite stage. Freeze-fracture replica showing a double row of nexus particles on the lateral wall of a myocardial plate cell.

Fig. 1.11. Freeze-fracture replica showing a small macular nexus on the lateral surface of a myocardial plate cell. The fracture plane has revealed both 'P' and 'E' faces at the nexus. Arrow in circle indicates direction of shadowing.

Fig. 1.12. Freeze-fracture replica showing a series of interconnected lines comprising tight junctions on the lateral wall of a myocardial plate cell near the pericardial lumen.

Fig. 1.13. Ninth day noon, 4-somite stage. Sagittal section showing the myocardial plate (M) bulging into the pericardial sac. H, headfold.

Fig. 1.14. Scanning electron micrograph of pericardial sac showing bilateral cardiac rudiments abutting against each other in the midline and delineated by a deep furrow. Photograph by courtesy of Professor M.H. Kaufman.

Fig. 1.15. Transmission electron micrograph showing superficial cells at the pericardial aspect (P) of the myocardial plate in a 4-somite stage embryo. These superficial cells contain typical striated myofibrillae and confirm that there is no distinct epicardial layer of cells.

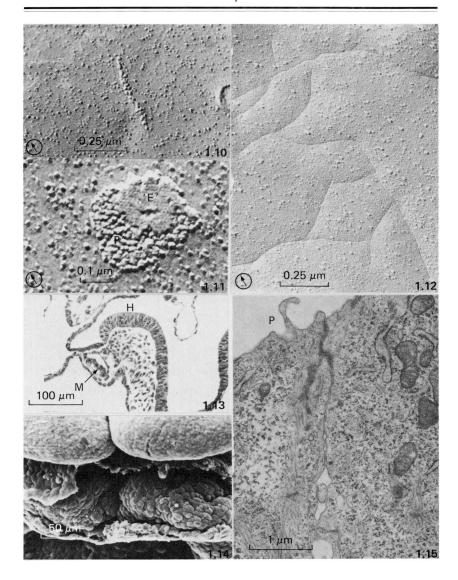

presumably occupied by cardiac jelly. As the endocardial rudiments and covering myocardial mantle progressively bulge into the peri-cardial sac, this is associated with a caudal movement of the intra-embryonic coelom. Because of this gradual relocation of the cardiac rudiment, the latter is now seen to be suspended by a wide 'mesocardium', the covering layer of which is continuous with the outer layer of myocardium.

The myocardium at this stage is composed of two or more cell layers throughout its extent and, though most of the outer layer of cells still retain their columnar orientation, the deeper cells have become more cuboidal or rounded in shape. There is no distinct epicardial layer covering the outer aspect of the myocardium; the most superficial myocardial cells, notwithstanding their columnar appearance and the presence of microvilli, resemble the deeper cells in cytoplasmic content including the presence of fascicles of fila-ments some of which are distinctly striated (Fig. 1.15).

The cytoplasm of myocardial cells is riddled with polysomes and monoribosomal granules though, probably because of the increase in filament content and mitochondria, they appear to be more diffusely distributed than before. There is a higher proportion of granules attached to the ER which itself has become more extensive. Most of the ER is of the granular variety though there are some smooth cisterns, similar to the sarcoplasmic reticulum (SR) of definitive myocardium, especially those situated subjacent to the cell surface. Of the large cytoplasmic organelles observed at this stage, mitochondria have perceptibly increased in number and there seem to be fewer electron-lucent droplets. Filaments are much more abundant than at previous stages, being dispersed throughout the cytoplasm, and fascicles of thin filaments (5–7 nm) were particu-larly frequently encountered near the sarcolemma (Fig. 1.15). There is evidence of transverse striation at regular intervals along these fascicles in the form of patches of electron-dense material, con-stituting the precursors of Z-lines; in addition there are thick filaments as well as thin filaments regularly interspersed within many fascicles. Some thin filaments are inserted into fasciae adherentes regions (interfibrillar or intermediate junctions) of the surface membrane near desmosomes.

With the formation of more than a single layer in the myocardial mantle, membrane apposition between cells has extended to include not only the lateral surface but also the other borders apart from those abutting the pericardial coelom. In addition, several small lacunar spaces are often seen between cells in the deeper part of the myocardium (Fig. 1.15) but no formed connective tissue elements, cellular or fibrous, are found in the intercellular space, so that it is unclear whether these spaces are the precursor sites of the fine capillaries that are found in similar locations at later stages.

An increase in gap junction contact between the myocytes compared to previous stages is also apparent and, in addition to the previously encountered punctate junctions, there are longer continuous stretches of close apposition. Ruthenium red labelling indicates the persistence of tight junctions between individual cells in the most superficial layer of the myocardium, but these cannot be discerned in the deeper layers of cells. Desmosomes are more numerous than at previous stages and interfibrillar junctions are also more extensive. However, there are no caveolae or T-tubule invaginations of the sarcolemma.

Freeze-fracture appearance

By this stage, it is relatively easy to locate the cardiac rudiment for freeze-fracture studies since both the pericardial sac and the myocardial mantle can be visualised under the low power magnification of a dissecting microscope.

In none of the replicas viewed can invaginations of the sarcolemma be found confirming that caveolae and T-tubules have not formed. Nexuses are, however, more readily identified at this stage not only because they are more extensive but also because the varied planes of membrane apposition render their exposure and replication easier. Linear arrays of nexus particles, circular annuli enclosing particle-free areas as well as maculae can be identified; some of the latter are fairly large in extent occasionally even exceeding 1 μm in diameter. Few tight junctions are encountered in the myocardium at this stage and, where present, they are restricted to the outermost cells abutting the pericardial sac.

Embryos with 5–6 pairs of somites

Between midday and early afternoon of the ninth day of pregnancy, most embryos are found to possess five or six pairs of somites. The cardiac rudiment is already slightly looped and asymmetrical, the bulbo-ventricular region being shifted slightly to the right of the midline and also ventrally into the pericardial coelom. Myocardial pulsations are readily elicited in many specimens; they seem to be fairly regular and are propagated from the caudal end of the rudiment towards its cranial end.

The scanning electron micrographs at this stage show that the median fissure between the primitive bilateral heart tubes becomes progressively filled out (see Kaufman & Navaratnam, 1981) and at about the six-somite stage, or slightly later, the ensuing single heart tube gradually folds to assume an S-shaped configuration.

Examination of semithin sections under the light microscope confirms that the endocardial rudiments have coalesced across the midline to establish a single continuous tube, the lumen of which shows a series of constrictions and dilatations. The heart tube is suspended into the pericardial cavity by a mesocardium that is now clearly dorsally located. The myocardial mantle comprises three or four layers of cells and the sub-endocardial space between the endocardial lining and the myocardium is wider than at any previous stage though it is still practically devoid of cells.

Examination of ultrathin sections reveals that the myocardial cells are irregular in shape with varying planes of contact and that striated myofibrillae are now conspicuously established in the cytoplasm (Fig. 1.16). There are numerous lacunae between cells but none of these are as yet lined by endothelium and there is no evidence of connective tissue cells or fibres or of neuronal elements. Over none of the myocardial sleeve has a separate epicardial layer differentiated; in Fig. 1.17, for example, a superficial myocardial cell is shown containing both myofilaments and microvilli at its pericardial aspect. Indeed, it is not till embryos with 12–15 pairs of somites are examined on the tenth day of pregnancy that separate flattened epicardial cells, lacking myofilaments, are found covering the superficial aspect of the myocardial sleeve (Fig. 1.18).

Surface invaginations of the sarcolemma such as caveolae or T-tubules have not yet developed and sub-sarcolemmal cisterns of SR still lack the structural specialisations usually associated with couplings of this type. Very rarely, vesicular profiles are found in the cytoplasm between myofibrillae but, in the absence of surface invaginations, these are more likely to be SR cisterns than T-tubules; in a single preparation, spherical vesicles are found near the sarcolemma (Fig. 1.16) but such an appearance is exceptional at this stage and there is no freeze-fracture evidence for the existence of caveolae (see p. 34). In general terms, the density of polysomes in the cytoplasm seems to have declined and the proportion of rough ER also appears less than before. In contrast there is considerable increase in myofibrillar content comprising fascicles of fine fila-ments interspersed with thick filaments (Fig. 1.16). These fascicles extend over relatively long distances, and they are interrupted at regular intervals by densities corresponding to the position of Z-lines but lacking their linear compactness. The orientation of myofibrillae is not entirely orderly, there being much branching and dispersal at various angles but, where a cell is elongated, the majority of its myofibrillae appear to be oriented along the same axis. Mitochondria have continued to increase in number and tend to be stacked between myofibrillae; their cristae are transversely aligned and closely packed. The few electron-lucent droplets present are interspersed among the mitochondria.

The varied planes of contact between myocardial cells sometimes facilitate the display of early step-like intercalated discs (Fig. 1.16) along which desmosomes, interfibrillar junctions and nexuses can be recognised. Most of the nexuses now comprise regions of membrane apposition over a substantial length (Fig. 1.17) and there are relatively few of the punctate variety still present.

Freeze-fracture appearance

Most of the material for freeze-fracture replication was derived
from the bulbo-ventricular region which is the most conspicuously
looped segment of the heart tube. Membrane surfaces are relatively
easy to find in the replicas and none of them show T-tubules or
caveolae. Nexuses are encountered fairly regularly and most of
them have assumed the form of macular patches. Many of the
maculae are relatively large, most exceeding 1 μm and some even
exceeding 2 μm in diameter. The junction particles are in general
closely packed in hexagonal fashion with a centre-to-centre spacing
of 10–12 nm but there are also narrow sinuous particle-free areas or
aisles within each patch. Few, if any, tight junctions are
encountered in the myocardium at this stage or later.

Résumé of differentiation on the eighth and ninth days of gestation

*Gross morphology and cellular differentiation of the heart
rudiment*

The foregoing account shows that myocardial cells differentiate as a
thickening of part of the splanchnic pericardial lining at the
presomite stage of development and subsequently elongate with
their apical surfaces directly exposed to the pericardial lumen, while

Fig. 1.16. Myocardium in a 6-somite stage embryo, isolated on the
evening of the ninth day. Note the varying planes of contact
between myocytes including numerous adherent-type junctions.
There are a few spherical vesicles near the sarcolemma but such
an appearance is unusual at this stage.

Fig. 1.17. Six-somite stage. An electron micrograph to show cells
at the pericardial surface (P) of the myocardial plate. These cells
contain myofibrillae confirming that there is no distinct epicardial
layer at this stage. There are fairly long stretches of nexus contact
between apposed myocardial cells.

Fig. 1.18. Electron micrograph of the myocardial sleeve of a
15-somite stage embryo, showing a non-myocytic epicardial cell
overlying the myocardial layer (M).

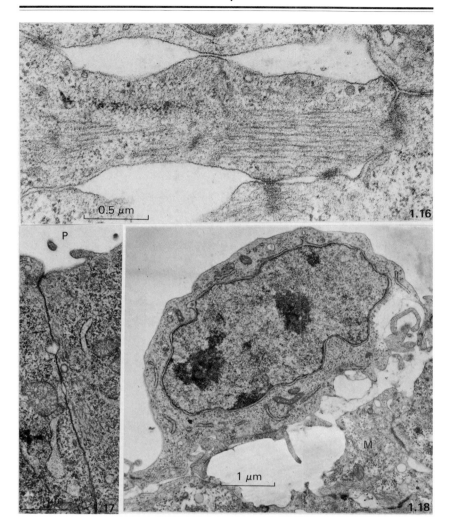

their basal surfaces overlie separate endocardial elements. The space between the latter elements and the myocardium subsequently widens, presumably to accommodate acellular cardiac jelly although the components of this substance could not be recognised in the present study. In addition to numerous ribosomes and other cytoplasmic organelles, such as mitochondria and glycogen granules, the cells of the myocardial plate at this stage contain large numbers of electron-lucent droplets which originate at the periphery of the Golgi apparatus and seem to enlarge in association with increased local ribosome activity. The droplets migrate to the periphery and their proximity to the cell membrane when mature suggests that they probably discharge their contents to the exterior. It is possible that the contents of these droplets may contribute to the formation of sub-endocardial cardiac jelly which is thought to develop about this time at the base of the myocardial plate but their more frequent association with the apical surface suggests the alternative idea that they contribute to the fluid contents of the pericardial sac thereby enlarging the latter.

With the formation of the myocardial plate the component cells divide mitotically and, during the ninth day, the plate becomes several layers thick with the cells contacting each other in different planes. As the heart tube enlarges, it progressively bulges into the pericardial cavity and is covered by a sleeve of myocardial cells which is complete except on the dorsolateral aspects where it is continuous with the endothelial lining of the pericardial coelom enclosing the dorsal mesocardium. Throughout the ninth day there is no distinct layer of epicardium covering the myocardium and there is no evidence of endothelially lined capillaries in the latter.

The 8–9-day period is one of enormous growth of the heart tube and its linear dimensions increase by a factor of four or five (Challice & Virágh, 1973), dextral looping occurs, the embryonic cardiac chambers become recognisable and the blood circulation is established at this time. Sissman (1970) claimed that the circulation starts on the eighth day of gestation but the dating of his material is not clear. In the present series the embryonic heart shows evidence of pulsation by about the 3–4-somite stage, i.e. during the morning of the ninth day of pregnancy, initially in a weak and irregular fashion but gradually strengthening to produce regular peristaltic contractions. At this time, the myocardium comprises a stratified sleeve of developing myocytes abutting each other, without any connective tissue elements, capillaries or neuronal processes. The myocytes are already equipped with striated myofibrillae, containing thick and thin filaments as well as segmentally arranged regions of electron density which subsequently condense into Z-lines. On the other hand, T-tubules and caveolae have not yet formed nor are the SR couplings with the sarcolemma clearly demarcated at this stage; cisterns of SR were frequently observed in typical sub-sarcolemmal positions but the cytoplasmic densities and intraluminal granules associated with definitive SR couplings (see Ayettey & Navaratnam, 1978a) could not be identified even in embryos possessing 5–6 pairs of somites.

Cell junctions in the developing myocardium

Following its differentiation from the wall of the pericardial coelom, the myocardial plate appears to be provided with recognisable albeit primitive junctional complexes *ab initio*. By the time that the pericardial cavity appears at the late presomite stage, the lining cells are seen to abut against each other along their lateral borders and there are clearly defined adherent-type junctions closely resembling desmosomes present. The earliest junctional complexes are situated near the pericardial lumen and, by the 1–2-somite stage, tight junctions and punctate nexuses can also be recognised. The tight junctions, which were revealed by ruthenium red labelling and by freeze-fracture replication, probably serve the purpose of sealing the pericardial sac by preventing its contents from escaping between the myoblasts. In comparison, Legato (1979) did not find specialised junctions in the myocardium of dog embryos until later stages of development.

The earliest nexuses are also formed between the apical parts of the myoblasts very near the tight junctions and desmosomes. Initially the nexuses are restricted in extent to punctate spots but, as the myoblasts elongate and as the myocardial plate comes to resemble a simple monolayer of columnar epithelium, they extend to form a series of punctate nexuses and later to form more complex conformations along their lateral borders. Desmosomal contact also increases but tight junctions remain restricted and are not found in deeper parts of the myocardial epithelium.

There are two main ways in which the proteins (connexons) comprising gap junction particles may aggregate within particular areas of cell membrane; they may either be inserted directly into a preformed junctional area of membrane or they may be inserted into any part of the membrane and then reach the junction by lateral movement. The latter mode is more likely because the former would require special mechanisms for the recognition of junctional membrane at the point of protein insertion (Loewenstein, 1981). Connexons or their subunits after insertion into the cell membrane probably move laterally at random till they come within range of attractive forces of apposing membranes. They then could interlock with reciprocal particles on the other membrane, become immobilised and establish an intercellular channel. When the apposition of myoblasts in the mouse myocardial plate is viewed in this light, it seems likely that the desmosome and tight junction apposition at the apices of these cells provides stable membrane apposition thus creating a trap leading to the linking of connexons. The initial site and extent of accretion of gap junction particles will be so determined but, as Loewenstein points out, the extent of the junction can increase as connexon pairing proceeds.

In the present study of the embryonic mouse myocardial plate, observations on thin sections and freeze-fracture replicas indicate that punctate and linear nexuses are initially established near co-existing tight junctions and desmosomes, reflecting a narrow zone of membrane apposition. Subsequently, the nexuses extend to form circular configurations as well as maculae of increasing size (see also Gros, Mocquard, Challice & Schrevel, 1978; Virágh & Challice, 1973). The extent of nexuses is enhanced by the increase in membrane contact area brought about as the myoblasts divide in various planes. Similarly the membrane apposition is further stabilised by an increase in the number of desmosomes and by the appearance of extensive fasciae adherentes, which, in turn, will allow the establishment of further nexuses. Kordylewski, Goings, Karrison & Page (1985) found in chick embryos that P-face particle density on cardiac myoblast plasma membranes increases rapidly on the third day of incubation, indicating a spurt of insertion of channel-, carrier- and receptor-proteins during the early somite period of embryogenesis.

Differentiation after the ninth day
Tenth day of gestation

Enlargement of the heart tube accelerates on the tenth day with increased looping especially ventrally into the pericardial cavity. The bulbo-ventricular and sinu-atrial chambers are recognisable under the dissecting microscope but there are no identifiable differences in myocardial ultrastructure between the various chambers.

Other developments on the tenth day, in embryos containing 12–15 pairs of somites, include the appearance for the first time of flattened epicardial cells lacking myofilaments (Fig. 1.18) on the superficial aspect of the myocardial sleeve and of caveolae in relation to the sarcolemma of many cardiac myocytes. Epicardial cells first appear on the dorsal aspect of the heart tube, where the dorsal mesocardium is currently undergoing fenestration to form the transverse pericardial sinus, suggesting that cells of the pericardial lining migrate from this site to form a complete covering. Lack of similarity, in both shape and cytoplasmic content, indicate that the early epicardial cells do not arise by de-differentiation of underlying myocytes. The present observations on mouse embryos support those of Manasek (1969) on the chick that epicardial cells arise from a source other than the myocardium. Capillaries are not present in the myocardial coat of 10-day embryos; however, as in younger embryos, there are numerous lacunae between cells which probably represent precursors of capillaries although they lack an endothelial lining.

As indicated above, caveolae have appeared in relation to the surface membrane of many myocytes. They mainly take the form of rounded invaginations of the membrane and, occasionally, there is fusion of adjacent vesicles which share a single mouth. No T-tubules can be identified but there are several superficial cisterns of SR coupled with the surface sarcolemma and some of these cisterns show intraluminal granules characteristic of junctional SR (Ayettey & Navaratnam, 1978a; Sommer & Johnson, 1979). There is no evidence of membrane-bound electron-dense granules resembling the specific granules of definitive atrial myocytes nor are there electron-lucent lipid droplets at this stage of development.

11–14 days gestation

By the twelfth day, the definitive positions of the various cardiac chambers have more or less been established by looping of the heart; the bulbo-ventricular chambers have shifted to lie caudal to the bulky atrium, from which they are demarcated by a narrow atrioventricular canal, and the sinus venosus has shifted towards the right on the dorso-caudal aspect of the atrium. During the next few days, part of the sinus venosus is absorbed into the dorsal atrial wall and internal partition of the cardiac chambers into systemic and pulmonary streams is effected. Both atrial and ventricular myocardium have essentially similar cell components but some distinguishing features can be recognised at this stage; for instance, intercellular lacunae are more prominent in the ventricular myocardium than in the atrium. Nerve axon profiles can be identified in the heart wall for the first time on or about the twelfth day and they are initially restricted to the sinu-atrial region. The early innervation of the venous side of the heart, compared to the arterial end, resembles the sequence observed in human embryos at about the 11-mm stage (Navaratnam, 1965b). By the fourteenth day nerve fibres have invaded the arterial end as well, near the base of the truncus arteriosus, but innervation of the atria remains more profuse and contains more numerous ganglion cells.

The epicardium has extended to form a continuous covering of the heart by the twelfth day and material labelled with ruthenium red shows that this layer is sealed with tight junctions. By the

fourteenth day, capillary spaces lined by a single layer of endothelium have appeared in the ventricular wall. The intercellular
space also contains occasional non-myocytic cells, possibly
fibroblasts, but there is no collagen in the region. Cell junctions in
the myocardium have assumed complex zig-zag patterns and they
include numerous desmosomes, nexuses and interfibrillar junctions
but no tight junctions.

The most conspicuous components of cardiac myocytes are
myofibrillae and mitochondria which together occupy about half
the cell volume. The myofibrillae are more regularly arranged than
before; the Z-lines have become compact and are in register in
several places. However, the arrangement is still not as compact as
in the adult there being plenty of loose cytoplasm containing
glycogen, ribosomes and SR. The mitochondria tend to be arranged
in columns between myofibrillae.

Myocytes at this stage are characterised by numerous caveolae
and by the fourteenth day some ventricular myocytes also contain a
few elongated invaginations resembling narrow T-tubules (Fig.
1.19). This observation of T-tubules in embryonic myocytes is at
variance with most other descriptions which indicate that they
appear only after the tenth day of postnatal life in the mouse
(Challice & Virágh, 1973) and in the rat (Hirakow, Gotoh &
Watanabe, 1980); however, a recent study by Forbes, Hawkey &
Sperelakis (1984) shows the presence of T-tubules in the ventricular
muscle of newborn mice. Initially, the T-tubules have a meandering
course and exhibit no couplings with SR at this stage; typical
couplings with junctional SR are restricted to the surface
sarcolemma.

Occasional droplets of electron-lucent material without a limiting membrane are found in the cytoplasm of a few myocytes, mainly
in the ventricular myocardium, and they are similar in appearance
to lipid droplets of the definitive myocardium. Smaller granules
(50–100 nm in diameter) enclosed by membrane and containing
electron-dense material are found near the maturing face of the
Golgi apparatus in both atrial and ventricular myocytes. They are
few in number and, although they resemble specific atrial granules

in some respects (see Challice & Virágh, 1973), their diminutive size and acid phosphatase content suggest that they are primary lysosomes. Evidence of lysosomal activity can be detected in the presence of occasional larger secondary lysosomes of the size of mitochondria, containing distorted cristae in the matrix. These features suggest that already mitochondria are being degraded and turned over.

Fifteenth day of gestation to the first postnatal day

During this period there is considerable growth of the heart with concomitant enlargement of myocytes which continues after birth to the neonatal period when ventricular myocytes become much larger than their atrial counterparts. A similar sequence of differential growth of ventricular and atrial myocytes has been observed in the neonatal rat by Hirakow, Gotoh & Watanabe (1980).

Fig. 1.19. Electron micrograph of ventricular myocyte in 14-day mouse foetus showing a T-tubule invagination (T) with luminal coating of basement membrane.

Fig. 1.20. Left atrial myocyte from 15-day mouse foetus showing a cluster of membrane-bound granules (g) near the Golgi apparatus.

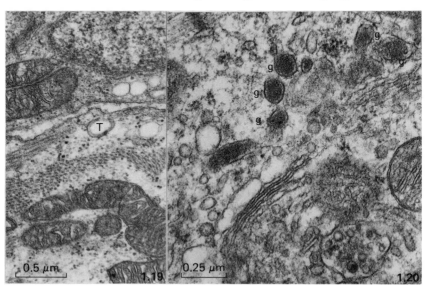

However, up to and including the first day after birth there is no difference in myocyte size between left and right atria and between left and right ventricles. Enlargement of myocytes during the terminal part of gestation is accompanied by exaggeration of myofibrillar content which occupies almost half the cell volume at birth. Fractional mitochondrial volume also increases substantially over the same period and undoubtedly continues to increase after birth (Sheridan, Cullen & Tynan, 1978). Other noticeable features of development include an increase in size and number of T-tubules especially in ventricular cells, but the T-system at birth is still restricted to primary invaginations unlike the elaborate network of primary, secondary and longitudinal elements in definitive cardiac myocytes. A few SR couplings are found in relation to primary T-tubules but peripheral SR couplings with the sarcolemma remain more numerous till after birth.

Apart from the small membrane-bound lysosomes, granules of a larger size (250–400 nm in diameter) containing electron-dense material have appeared near the Golgi apparatus and nuclear poles by the fifteenth day of gestation (Fig. 1.20) and positive labelling with colloidal gold conjugated with antibody to atriopeptin 28 can be detected. They are more prevalent in atrial myocytes but a few are found in ventricular cells as well. In the neonatal material, their numbers have increased substantially in atrial cells where they can be found not only near the nucleus but also further out in the cytoplasm scattered among mitochondria and occasionally near the sarcolemma. Their immunoreactivity to atriopeptin is fairly heavy by this stage. The appearance of such atrial specific granules could represent a preparatory step prior to birth, after which the neonatal pup would be required to cope independently with electrolyte and fluid balance. The number of granules in ventricular cells falls off and becomes negligible at birth. Moreover, although myocytes in most parts of the atrial wall contain such granules, it is noticeable that cells in the sinu-atrial region of the right atrium contain few or none.

Lipid droplets are also more numerous than at previous stages but, unlike specific granules, they are mainly restricted to ventricular myocytes in which they lie scattered among the mitochondrial columns.

―――

Formation of the presumptive pericardial cavity in mouse embryos commences during the late presomite stage (afternoon of the eighth day) and the myocardial rudiment originates *in situ* as a thickening of the splanchnic pericardial lining. Initially, the myocardium comprises an epithelium directly exposed to the pericardial lumen and overlying a separate layer of endocardial elements. As the heart bulges into the pericardial coelom, it becomes surrounded by a sleeve of myocardium which thickens and stratifies during the ninth day and later, on the tenth day (about the 15-somite stage), it acquires an epicardial lining of flattened cells.

The myocardium commences pulsations at about the 3–4-somite stage (morning of the ninth day) by which time it can be shown by transmission electron microscopy that the myoblasts already contain striated myofibrillae and specialised cell junctions. From its earliest appearance, the myocardial plate contains tight junctions and desmosomes between the lateral borders of the myoblasts near their apical ends and the junctional complexes are impermeable to ruthenium red. Freeze-fracture replicas show that nexuses soon appear in the same region and that they increase in number and extent, as the myoblasts elongate and divide; they are supplemented by the formation of interfibrillar junctions and more desmosomes while tight junctions decline in extent and are eventually confined to the epicardium.

By the twelfth day, the epicardium has extended to form a continuous covering of the heart and by the fourteenth day capillary vessels lined by endothelium can be recognised in the ventricular wall. About the same time, rudimentary T-tubules appear in cardiac myocytes which by now also include a few lipid droplets and primary lysosomes containing acid phosphatase activity. Granules which are immunoreactive for atriopeptin appear about the fifteenth day and they increase in number and immunoreactivity in atrial myocytes during the late prenatal and early neonatal periods.

2

Ultrastructure of typical myocardial cells

Typical myocardium is built up of more-or-less cylindrical, elongated and branched myocytes containing a centrally placed nucleus (for a summary of myocardial cell alignment see Sommer, 1982). The surface membrane at the ends of each cell is apposed to that of its neighbours forming intercalated discs which include specialised junctions. The size of component myocytes varies according to the region of the heart, being thickest in the general ventricular myocardium (in the rat the average ventricular cell has a diameter of about 16 μm and a length of about 105 μm) while cells in the atrial myocardium are more slender and elongated (11 μm in diameter and 127 μm in length). The sinu-atrial and atrioventricular nodes contain the smallest cells (about 6 μm in diameter and 45 μm in length) while the size of myocytes in the atrioventricular bundle and its branches depends on the species. In most species including the mouse, golden hamster, cat, rat, dog and man, myocytes in the bundle system are relatively small ranging in size between nodal cells and typical ventricular cells. On the other hand, in ungulates and cetaceans, bundle cells are larger than those of the general myocardium (Caesar, Edwards & Ruska, 1958; Hayashi, 1962) and cells in the peripheral ramifications of the bundle are even larger thus resembling typical Purkinje cells.

In this account attention is focussed mainly on the features of typical ventricular myocardial cells but it also includes comments on the contrasting features of other cardiac myocytes.

Nucleus

The nuclei of cardiac myocytes do not present many distinctive features when compared with nuclei of other cells. They are usually irregular in outline with occasional deep indentations which may simulate the appearance of multiple nuclei; however, close analysis shows that cells with more than a single nucleus are very rare (Simpson, Rayns & Ledingham, 1973). In material initially fixed with aldehydes and postfixed with osmium tetroxide, the nuclear chromatin is evenly dispersed so that condensations of nuclear material, apart from one or two nucleoli, are infrequent. The nuclear membrane forms a double-layered envelope, as in other cells, and the interstice between its component layers communicates with that of the sarcoplasmic reticulum. The outer surface of the nuclear membrane is generally smooth but does bear some scattered ribosomes. Numerous nuclear pores are seen in sectioned material and in freeze-fracture replicas (Fig. 2.1).

There have been occasional descriptions of distinctive features of the nucleus in cardiac myocytes. For example, Fawcett & McNutt (1969) have described small outpocketings of the nuclear envelope adjacent to Golgi complexes in the cat myocardium but these have not been confirmed by other investigators. More encouraging are the recent observations on freeze-fracture preparations of rabbit myocardium reported by Severs (1984). Using filipin labelling as a cholesterol probe, he observed that the nuclear envelope in cardiac myocytes is unlabelled, unlike capillary endothelial cells where the nuclear envelope contains identifiable cholesterol albeit less than in the plasma membrane. A satisfactory explanation for this difference has not yet been advanced, though it is possible that the failure of filipin labelling is caused by differences in physical features of the nuclear membrane affecting access to cholesterol in cardiac myocytes rather than by differences in membrane chemistry.

Sarcolemma

The plasma membrane in all varieties of cardiac myocytes has the features of a typical unit membrane and it measures about 8–9 nm in thickness. It is closely associated with a basement membrane or laminar coat which has a layered appearance comprising a flocculent electron-dense zone of about 30 nm separated by an electron-lucent interval of about 20 nm from the outer surface of the sarcolemma (Sommer & Johnson, 1979). The flocculent layer gives attachment to collagen fibrils which lie further out in the extracellular space (Fig. 2.2). Cytochemical data indicate that the laminar coat contains polyanionic groups including carbohydrate-containing material such as proteoglycans and the glycoproteins, fibronectin and laminin. However, in regions where there is close apposition between myocytes, sugar residues are reduced and the laminar coat is attenuated and difficult to recognise (Gros & Challice, 1975) unless stained with a substance such as ruthenium red which enhances the electron density of basement membrane material.

The plasma membrane of cardiac myocytes is characterised by numerous invaginations principally caveolae, which are present in all varieties, and T-tubules which are prominent in the general myocardium but sparse in nodal cells (see Chapter 4). Other features of the cell membrane include specialised cell junctions

Fig. 2.1. Freeze-fracture replica of adult guinea-pig left ventricle showing part of the nuclear membrane (N) with numerous pores, surface sarcolemma (S) with T-tubule openings (T) and caveolae (arrows) and the intervening cytoplasm containing mitochondria (M) and a series of primary T-tubules (T). Arrow in circle indicates direction of shadowing.

Fig. 2.2. Thin section of left atrial myocardium in adult rat, showing typical basement membrane of cardiac myocytes comprising a flocculent electron-dense zone (arrow) separated from the plasma membrane by an electron-lucent interval. Note the cistern of junctional sarcoplasmic reticulum (SR) containing luminal granules and coupled with surface sarcolemma. v, coated vesicle.

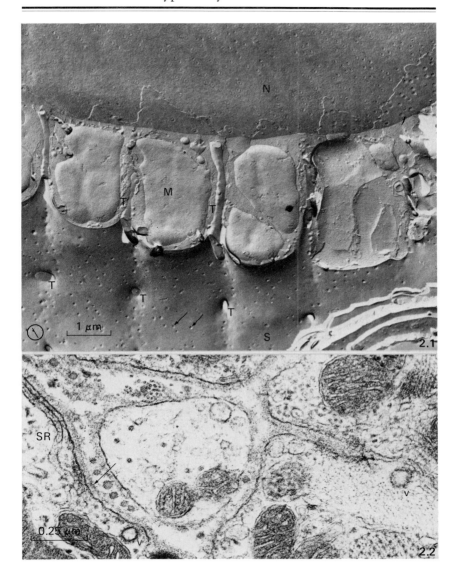

which are typically grouped at intercalated discs (see p. 36) and
numerous couplings with the sarcoplasmic reticulum.

Cytochemical investigations using Pb^{2+} as capture ions have
demonstrated the presence of adenylate cyclase and guanylate
cyclase along the plasma membrane (Schultze, 1984). Regarding
ATPases, Pb^{2+}-capture techniques have shown the presence of a
'basic' ATPase (it has a broad pH maximum from 7.0 to 10.0) on
the cytoplasmic aspect of the membrane (Malouf & Meissner,
1984) but the functional significance of this enzyme is uncertain.
Lead ions are not suitable for capturing (Na^+K^+) ATPase because
they have a strong inhibitory effect, but the use of Sr^{2+} has been of
limited success in demonstrating this enzyme along the plasma
membrane though the localisation has not been precise. Cytochemical techniques indicate that $(Ca^{2+}Mg^{2+})$ ATPase is not present at
this site.

Caveolae

Caveolae are small (diameter about 50–80 nm) flask-shaped invaginations of the plasma membrane accompanied by basement
membrane on the luminal surface. They are found at the surface of
the cell including parts of intercalated discs and, to a lesser extent,
along T-tubule invaginations. They communicate with the extracellular space or T-tubule lumen by way of a slightly constricted neck
and the openings can be visualised either in thin sections (Fig. 2.2)
or in freeze-fracture preparations (Fig. 2.1). Sometimes, multiple
caveolae (up to five have been observed) communicate with a single
neck. The lumen may contain granular material and the intensity of
labelling after administration of horseradish peroxidase indicates
ready interchange with the extracellular space. Although some
authors have described indications of orderliness in the positions of
caveolae on the surface of cardiac myocytes (see Sommer &
Johnson, 1979, for review), the general view is that the distribution
is random. Caveolae are more numerous on the surface of atrial
myocytes than that of ventricular cells and it has been suggested
that they are most frequent in cells lacking a T-system (Forssmann
& Girardier, 1970).

Though they undoubtedly increase the surface area, the functions of the caveolae in cardiac myocytes are unknown. They have not been demonstrated to have a pinocytotic function and Essner, Novikoff & Quintana (1965) found that they differ from pinocytotic vesicles of capillary endothelium in lacking ATPase activity. Caveolae do not form coupling arrangements with the sarcoplasmic reticulum (SR).

Other surface vesicles

Coated pits and coated vesicles have been observed in all varieties of cardiac myocytes. They are much less frequent than caveolae, slightly larger (80–100 nm in diameter), and possess a coat of fine radiating bristles on their cytoplasmic aspect (Fig. 2.2); by analogy with coated vesicles elsewhere, the bristles are thought to contain clathrin and the vesicles are thought to mediate protein transport. Such vesicles may communicate with the surface of the cell or with T-tubules or, unlike caveolae, they may be found deep in the cytoplasm near the Golgi apparatus or in contact with sarcoplasmic reticulum.

T-tubule system

Both freeze-fracture replicas and thin-sectioned material indicate that there is some orderliness in the arrangement of primary T-tubule invaginations, in comparison with caveolae (Fig. 2.1). Rows of openings occur at about Z-line level from which the tubules extend towards the myofibrillar I-bands on either side of the Z-line. Within the sarcoplasm, the primary tubules lead to a branching system (Fig. 2.3), the extent of which varies according to the region of myocardium (see Chapter 4 for details and for a review of the literature); in ventricular myocardium the T-tubule system is elaborately branched and it has numerous couplings with the SR.

The appearance of the unit membrane of T-tubules closely resembles that of the surface sarcolemma in thin sections and in freeze-fracture material. Moreover, cytochemical studies indicate that the localisation of adenylate cyclase and guanylate cyclase (Schultze, 1984) and that of ATPases (Butcher, 1983; Malouf &

Meissner, 1984) of the T-tubule membrane resemble those at the surface plasma membrane. In other words, the T-tubule membrane system represents a second (internal) system of plasma membrane which complicates the electrical behaviour of the muscle fibre (Sommer & Johnson, 1979).

Intercalated discs

Even under the light microscope, thickened densities differing from Z-lines can be discerned across the long axis of muscle fibres. Before the advent of the electron microscope these were generally assumed to constitute intracellular structures though Eberth (1866) ventured the view that they constitute intercellular cement substance. Early electron microscope studies by van Breemen (1953), Sjöstrand & Andersson (1954) and Muir (1957) established that the so-called

Fig. 2.3. Diagram showing some cytoplasmic features of a typical cardiac myocyte. The T-tubule system (T) comprises primary invaginations of the sarcolemma which give off secondary transverse branches as well as longitudinal branches. The longitudinal branches are further linked by narrow tertiary transverse tubules at A-band level. At all levels of the T-system there occur couplings with cisterns of sarcoplasmic reticulum (SR). Superficial couplings of SR with the surface sarcolemma are also present. Myofibrillae contain thin filaments, which are attached to Z-lines, and thick filaments which occupy the A-band region of each sarcomere; there is partial overlap of these filaments giving the typical striated appearance of myofibrillae.

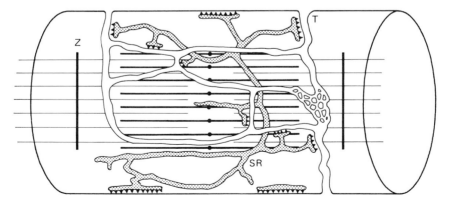

intercalated discs are in fact junctional complexes comprising
apposition and specialisation of the sarcolemma of adjacent myocardial cells. Detailed ultrastructural features of the intercalated
disc have since been described by several authors including
Sjöstrand, Andersson-Cedergren & Dewey (1958), Dewey (1969),
Kawamura & James (1971) and Staehelin (1974).

A typical intercalated disc has a step-wise or undulant
appearance with alternating transverse and lateral segments (Figs.
2.4, 2.5, 2.6). The transverse components of a disc always occur at
the end of a sarcomere replacing the Z-line at that level. Each disc
may contain up to four types of junctions: (1) nexuses (also termed
gap junctions or communicating junctions); (2) desmosomes
(maculae adherentes) of the circumscribed or spot variety; (3)
interfibrillar junctions (also termed intermediate junctions or
fasciae adherentes) which constitute the regions of myofilament
insertion; (4) apparently unspecialised regions. Of these junctions,
nexuses always occupy the lateral components of the disc, i.e. they
run parallel with the long axis of the fibre, interfibrillar junctions lie
transverse to the long axis, while desmosomes and structurally

Fig. 2.4. Diagram showing the components of a typical
intercalated disc. D, desmosome; N, nexus; I, interfibrillar or
intermediate junction. The remainder of the disc is apparently
unspecialised and shows features of the surface sarcolemma
elsewhere including couplings with cisterns of sarcoplasmic
reticulum (SR).

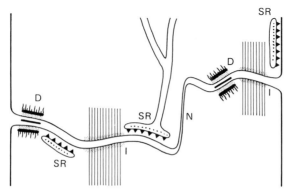

unspecialised components may occupy any part of a disc. Over most of the disc, the gap between apposed membranes is about 20–25 nm but it is reduced to about 2 nm along nexus components. There are no tight junctions (maculae occludentes) in the adult myocardium although they are present as a transient feature in the early embryonic myocardial plate (Chapter 1). Prominent inter-calated discs containing all four components are characteristically present in the general atrial and ventricular myocardium and in the atrioventricular bundle system but the nodes contain inconspicuous cell junctions (Fig. 2.7) mainly comprising apposition of unspecial-ised membrane reinforced by occasional desmosomes and punctate nexuses.

Nexuses, which are composed of protein channels between the cytoplasmic compartments of adjacent cells, are described in detail in Chapter 3 where the relevant literature also is reviewed. The basement membrane is excluded or very inconspicuous in the narrowed labyrinthine space at nexus components and the apposed plasma membranes are not associated with caveolae, SR couplings, fibrillar insertions or other features generally associated with sur-face sarcolemma. Indeed the zones of sarcoplasm adjacent to each nexus are relatively free of cytoplasmic organelles though the immediate inner aspect of the membrane may be coated with fuzzy material. The plasma membranes at nexuses possess cyclase activity (Schultze, 1984) but lack cytochemically demonstrable ATPase (Malouf & Meissner, 1984).

As in other tissues, desmosomes in the myocardium are assumed

Fig. 2.5. Electron micrograph of left atrial myocardium from adult rat to show components of an intercalated disc. N, nexus on a longitudinal segment of the disc; I, intermediate junction. Note couplings between sarcolemma at an unspecialised region of the disc with cisterns of junctional sarcoplasmic reticulum (arrows).

Fig. 2.6. Freeze-fracture replica of left ventricular myocardium from adult ferret showing an intercalated disc including a nexus (arrow) on a longitudinal segment. The plane of fracture has revealed both 'P' and 'E' faces of membrane at the region of the nexus.

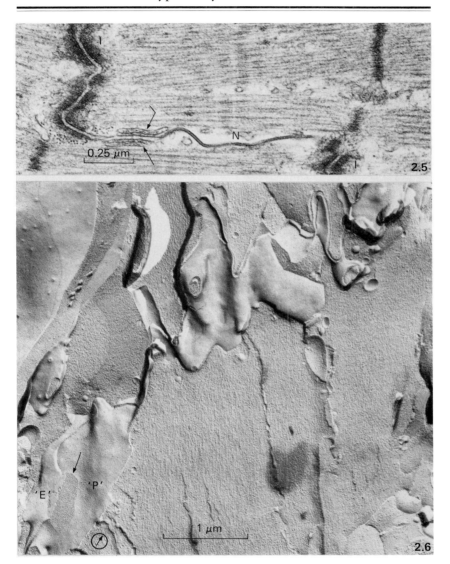

to serve the function of cell-to-cell adhesion. The adhesive spots range in size from 200 to 400 nm in diameter and each junction comprises apposed membranes separated by a gap of 20–25 nm. These membranes are not associated with caveolae, SR couplings or myofilament insertion and they show 'basic' ATPase activity. On the cytoplasmic aspect of each membrane, there are thickened plaques into which tonofilaments (about 10 nm in diameter) insert (Figs. 2.4, 2.7). The intercellular gap between the membranes lodges a median line of considerable density which has been shown by sections in appropriate planes to comprise a zig-zag structure with lateral extensions. The density is a specialisation of the basement membrane comprising glycoproteins and the integrity of the bond is dependent on Ca^{2+}.

Interfibrillar or intermediate junctions occur at levels where a Z-line would normally be expected and they provide attachment for actin myofilaments. The apposed membranes are separated by a gap of 20–30 nm and, on their cytoplasmic aspects, there is a zone of increased density containing a feltwork of fibrillar material not dissimilar in appearance to Z-band material and probably composed of α-actinin and desmin. A central dense line can be discerned in the space between the apposed membranes and, although it is much less conspicuous than the corresponding density in desmosomes, it seems similarly to depend on Ca^{2+} for its integrity as EDTA removal of calcium causes their separation.

The membranes at the structurally unspecialised regions of the

Fig. 2.7. Thin sections to show cell junctions in sinu-atrial node region of golden hamster. There are few, if any, intercalated discs and the junctions mainly comprise desmosomes (D).

Fig. 2.8. Electron micrograph of rat atrial myocardium to show features of myofibrillae. Each sarcomere comprises the length between consecutive Z-lines and includes A-bands, containing thick filaments, and I-bands from which thick filaments are excluded. Thin filaments, which are attached on either side of Z-lines pass through the I-bands and overlap the thick filaments in the A-bands. The middle of each A-band shows an M-line of increased density flanked by lighter H-zones representing the region where thin filaments are absent. g, atrial specific granules.

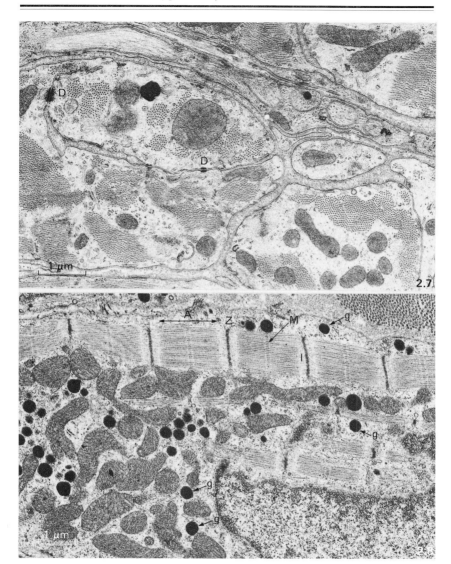

intercalated disc are very similar to the plasma membrane at the surface of the myocyte. The intercellular gap is reduced to 20–30 nm and basement membrane material is attenuated or even imperceptible in places. There are caveolae, but not T-tubule invaginations, and couplings with SR. Cytochemical staining shows the presence of adenylate cyclase and guanylate cyclase (Schultze, 1984) and 'basic' ATPase, though (Na^+K^+) ATPase has not been demonstrated at these sites.

Internal membrane systems

Sarcoplasmic reticulum

The sarcoplasmic reticulum (SR) forms an extensive network, the three-dimensional distribution of which can be visualised by high-voltage electron microscopy of comparatively thick sections (Peachey, Waugh & Sommer, 1974). It is not easy to distinguish from the T-tubule system without extracellular tracer labelling. The lumen of the SR is narrower than most of the T-system and it does not communicate with the extracellular space. Numerous couplings occur between the SR and plasma membrane (Figs. 2.2, 2.3, 2.5) or T-tubule membranes; the appearance of these couplings and their likely significance in the excitation-contraction sequence are considered in Chapter 4. Most of the SR is of the smooth variety though cisterns of granular SR are frequently found in developing cardiac myocytes (see Chapter 1). Cytochemical studies show that ($Ca^{2+}Mg^{2+}$) ATPase is localised at the SR membrane (Malouf & Meissner, 1984). This magnesium-dependent and calcium-activated enzyme is best demonstrated on unfixed tissue by a lead-capture technique but it is advisable to use a chelating agent to keep the concentration of Pb^{2+} sufficiently low.

Golgi apparatus

The Golgi apparatus is most pronounced in atrial myocytes where it is found close to the nuclear membrane both at the poles and alongside the length of the nucleus. Each stack comprises three to five flattened saccules and many small vesicles which are coated with a polyhedral lattice; some of the vesicles are clear but others, particularly those on the maturing or *trans* face which usually faces away from the nucleus, have electron-dense contents. Larger atrial granules (see Chapter 6) and primary lysosomes (Chapter 7) occur in the vicinity of the Golgi apparatus from which they probably arise.

The cisterns at the *trans* face of the Golgi apparatus are intensely positive for acid phosphatase (AP) and some positive elements are present in more peripheral situations. In ventricular myocytes, Golgi components are less extensive than in atrial cells and AP activity is less intense; nonetheless, they can be recognised both deep in the cytoplasm and near the periphery.

Contractile elements

The contractile apparatus of heart muscle as in skeletal muscle consists of (1) contractile proteins, i.e. myosin (which accounts for 60% of the myofibrillar mass) and actin (15%), (2) regulatory proteins, i.e. tropomyosin (10%) and troponins (5%), and (3) structural proteins (< 10%) including α-actinin, desmin and C-protein (Zak & Galhotra, 1983). The proteins of the three classes make up the myofibrils though, in heart muscle, the mass is only partially broken up into bundles of varying size by intersections of sarcoplasm containing mitochondria, SR, glycogen, lipid droplets and other organelles. Unlike skeletal muscles, there are no discrete myofibrils maintained as distinct organelles from one end of the cell to the other; the irregularity of myofibrillar material is especially pronounced in the myocytes of the sinu-atrial and atrioventricular nodes (Virágh & Porte, 1961*a,b*, 1973*a,b*; James & Sherf, 1968; Virágh & Challice, 1973; Taylor, 1980). The myofibrillar mass accounts for about half to two-thirds of the cell volume in working atrial and ventricular myocardium; it is less abundant in the majority of nodal cells but in some species there is appreciable variation in ultrastructural features, including myofibrillar content, among cells within the nodes and in the junctional myocardium adjacent to the nodes (Virágh & Porte, 1973*a,b*; Thaemert, 1973; Sommer, 1982).

In longitudinal section, cardiac muscle has a striated appearance like that of skeletal muscle reflecting a similar organisation of actin and myosin filaments. Light microscopy shows alternating light (isotropic or I) bands and dark (anisotropic or A) bands. The middle of each I-band is traversed by a Z-line and the region between two consecutive Z-lines constitutes a sarcomere which regularly repeats itself along the long axis of the cell; each sarcomere measures about 2.5 μm in relaxed muscle and about 1.5 μm in the contracted state. The A-bands remain constant in extent (about 1.5 μm) whereas the I-bands are variable, being longer in relaxation and practically disappearing during full contraction (see Spiro & Sonnenblick, 1964; Sonnenblick *et al.*, 1967). Detailed inspection reveals that each A-band is bisected by a dark M-line flanked on either side by a lighter H-zone (Fig. 2.8) but the latter is often only vaguely defined in cardiac muscle.

The characteristic banded appearance is determined by the arrangement of two main types of myofilaments (Fig. 2.3) namely (i) thick filaments (10–15 nm in diameter) which are composed of myosin and (ii) thin filaments (5–7 nm) which are mainly composed of actin but which also contain tropomyosin and troponin molecules. The A-band is co-extensive with the thick filaments. The thin filaments are attached to both sides of each Z-line and they extend so that their ends overlap parts of the thick filaments to which they are attached by cross-bridges within the A-bands; the lengths of thin filaments on either side of the Z-line which are not thus overlapped comprise the I-bands. The H-zone represents the region where thick filaments are not overlapped by thin filaments and the M-line is the site of localised thickenings of myosin filaments possibly augmented by cross-bridges in the vicinity. The imprecise appearance of the H-zone in heart muscle is probably attributable to the varied lengths of thin filaments causing a composite broad region of overlap with thick filaments.

The sliding filament hypothesis suggests that the fundamental contractile event in striated muscle is interaction between actin and myosin, comprising attachment and detachment of cross-bridges between thick and thin filaments which causes the thin filaments to slide along the thick filaments towards the centre of the A-band (Huxley, 1973). The result is the shortening of the muscle, or the generation of force during isometric phases when shortening is resisted. During relaxation, the regulatory proteins tropomyosin and troponin prevent reactions between actin and myosin but the inhibition is released when calcium ions are made available. The sliding filament hypothesis is based on evidence derived from skeletal muscle but the ultrastructural details of cardiac myocytes are compatible with its predictions.

Z-lines

In mammals, normal Z-lines are straight and of uniform width whereas in lower vertebrates they are wavy and less uniformly structured. Attempts have been made to analyse the geometry and chemical composition of the Z-line but, so far, these matters have not been completely elucidated. Most of the investigations have been conducted on skeletal muscle but Goldstein, Schroeter & Sass (1977) have studied the optical diffraction of the Z-lattice in canine heart muscle and Simpson, Rayns & Ledingham (1973) have considered to what extent it is feasible to extrapolate information from skeletal muscle to heart muscle. Longitudinal sections through the Z-line may show a number of appearances, and models have been proposed to explain these differences; at Z-line level, thin filaments may give way to a further type of filament or branch into subfilaments which may either pass into the next sarcomere, where they connect or interdigitate with thin filaments, or they may loop back to neighbouring thin filaments in the same sarcomere. Some of the problems of interpretation arise because the disposition of filament profiles within the Z-band depends on the method of fixation; for instance osmium fixation gives rise to a basket weave appearance while glutaraldehyde-osmium fixation produces a square lattice pattern.

Chemical analysis shows that actin is not a major component of the Z-band; on the other hand there is some evidence to indicate that it is mainly composed of α-actinin and desmin. The electron-dense material at the Z-line is in many ways similar to the dense material at the intermediate junctions of intercalated discs where thin filaments are inserted.

Myosin

The thick filaments composed of myosin have a diameter of 10–15 nm and a length of about 1.5 μm and they are set in a hexagonal pattern. Myosin is one of the largest proteins known, having a molecular weight of around 500 kD. Each molecule includes a dimer of heavy chains with dissimilar light chains attached to each strand. Details of the configuration of the molecule are provided by Zak & Galhotra (1983). Essentially each molecule is Y-shaped in which each arm comprises a globular head formed by the folded heavy chain and the stem comprises the intertwined helical region of the chains (Fig. 2.9). Cytochemical studies for ATPase have indicated the localisation of the reaction product at regular intervals/corresponding to myosin heads along the long axis of the A-band (Tice & Barnett, 1962; Sommer & Spach, 1964) and, more recently, Butcher (1983) described specific localisation of myosin ATPase at both light microscope and electron microscope levels without reaction in the sarcolemma, SR or mitochondria.

The myosin heads constitute the actin-binding or cross-bridging region in addition to possessing ATPase activity (Ebashi, 1963) and, in each sarcomere, they point away from the middle of the A-band (Fig. 2.9); the aggregation of molecules is such that successive pairs are separated by regular intervals of length and angular rotation. It is not yet known why the polarity of myosin molecules becomes reversed at the middle of the thick filament nor is it known how the molecules aggregate on each side of the M-line in such regular order.

Myosin does not exist as a single prototype molecule and several variants (isomyosins) exhibiting polymorphism of both heavy and light chains have been described. Two main classes of myosin have been described, one in fast skeletal muscle and the other in slow and cardiac muscles, but each class includes several sub-varieties. In the heart alone, the family of myosins is complex and cardiac myosin differs not only between species and individuals but also between regions in the same heart. For instance, atria and ventricles contain distinct sets of isomyosins which differ in the primary structure of heavy chains, type of light chains and in ATPase activity (Zak & Galhotra, 1983) and there appear to be further variations within each set.

The thick filaments are held together at their midpoints which collectively form the M-line (about 90 nm thick) across the middle of the A-band. At high magnification, the M-line can be resolved

Fig. 2.9. Diagrams showing the arrangement and configuration of thick filaments which are composed of myosin molecules. Each molecule is a dimer with globular heads and a stem comprising intertwined chains. The heads point away from the M-line at the middle of the A-band of each sarcomere and successive pairs are separated by regular intervals of length and angular rotation.

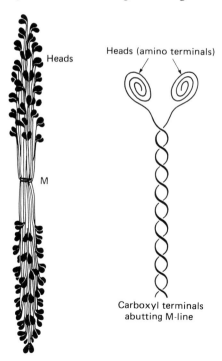

into three or five fine transverse lines (Fawcett & McNutt, 1969) which are thought to correspond to bridges between adjacent thick filaments (Simpson, Rayns & Ledingham, 1973).

Actin

Thin filaments, which are primarily composed of actin, have a diameter of 5–7 nm and a length of about 1 μm. The vast majority of these filaments in cardiac myocytes are found in the myofibrillar mass where they interdigitate with the thick filaments in such a way that each thick filament is surrounded by six thin filaments and each of these is situated at the trigonal point between three thick filaments. In addition, there have been descriptions especially in lower vertebrates (Sommer & Johnson, 1979) of microfilaments presumably composed of actin lying unoriented in the cytoplasm.

The monomer (G-actin) has a low molecular weight of about 45 kD but in myocytes, all actin exists in the polymerised (F-actin) form, and each thin filament contains two strands of actin wound round each other. In muscle contraction, the main functions of actin are to increase the activity of myosin ATPase and to interact with myosin. The interaction consists of attachment to the myosin head utilising the energy freed by ATP hydrolysis. Each actin monomer has two myosin-binding sites each of which is specific for different portions of the myosin head.

In comparison with myosin, actin exhibits a high degree of evolutionary conservation and there are only minor differences between actins from different varieties of cell in regard to molecular weight, activation of myosin ATPase or binding to myosin.

Tropomyosin

Tropomyosin is a polypeptide dimer forming a relatively rigid molecule which lies in the long pitched grooves on either side of the actin filament thereby stiffening the latter (Fig. 2.10); it is also closely bound to the troponin complex (see below). It has a molecular weight of about 65 kD and a length of 40 nm; the molecules are bonded head to tail, thereby forming a cable which spans the entire length of the thin filament. In the resting state, tropomyosin covers the myosin-binding sites of actin filaments. During activation, when the Ca^{2+} level is raised, the tropomyosin molecules are believed to shift allowing the myosin heads to interact with actin. The shift may be caused by alterations in the shape of the adjacent troponin molecules.

Two classes of tropomyosin exist: α and β (Zak & Galhotra, 1983). Most of the myocardial tropomyosin is of the α class resembling fast skeletal muscle, whereas heart muscle resembles slow muscle in many other properties such as the structure of myosin chains, speed of contraction and metabolic pattern. Pure α-tropomyosin is said to be typical of small mammals with fast heart rates (Leger, Bouveret, Schwartz & Swynghedauw, 1976), whereas

Fig. 2.10. Diagram showing the components of a thin filament.

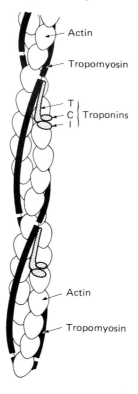

in the more slowly contracting hearts of large mammals a second band (possibly β-tropomyosin) is present.

Troponin

Troponin is a complex of three polypeptides (Troponins-T, -I and -C) which is localised at regular intervals along the thin filament, in close apposition to the tropomyosin chain (Fig. 2.10). The three components differ in their primary structure and have different functions. Troponin-T has a molecular weight of about 38 kD and readily forms complexes with tropomyosin and with troponin-C, thus anchoring the complex to the thin filament. Troponin-I has a molecular weight of about 27 kD and, when added to troponin-T and tropomyosin, it inhibits the interaction of actin and myosin even in the presence of Ca^{2+}. Troponin-C (18 kD) is a calcium ligand, capable of binding up to four Ca^{2+} though only two of these are high-affinity sites and of physiological significance. When Ca^{2+} is so bound, the configuration of the troponin complex is thought to be so altered as to shift the tropomyosin molecule off the myosin-binding sites on the thin filaments.

The variant of troponin-C present in cardiac muscle differs from that in fast muscles but is believed to be very similar or even identical to that in slow muscles (Wilkinson, 1980). Differences have also been described between the varieties of troponin-T and -I in fast, slow and cardiac muscles (Syska, Perry & Trayer, 1974; Dhoot & Perry, 1979) but the functional significance of such differences is not yet understood.

Mitochondria

Cardiac muscle, especially ventricular myocardium, is rich in mitochondria which occupy 20–40% of cell volume (Schaper, Meiser & Stämmler, 1985, and see Table 5.1) reflecting the high metabolic demand imposed by the repetitive cardiac cycle; the proportional volume occupied by mitochondria is particularly high among small mammals with a rapid heart rate and in bats which require adaptations for long periods of flight. Though myocardial mitochondria (Fig. 2.11) have similar ultrastructural components to mitochondria elsewhere, their cristae tend to be more tightly packed and to have a more regular transverse orientation whilst their matrix is reduced; consequently, the proportion of inner membrane area to outer membrane area is strikingly high. Electron-dense matrix granules have been observed in cardiac mitochondria especially in atrial myocytes (Armiger & Benson, 1978) and immunocytochemical studies indicate that they are associated with cytochrome oxidase (Hertsens, Bernaert, Jonian & Jacob, 1986); more granules, not necessarily of similar nature, appear after ischaemic damage (Kloner, Fishbein, Hare & Maroko, 1979, and see Chapter 5). Mitochondria in nodal myocytes are proportionately less numerous than in the general myocardium and their cristae are more loosely and irregularly arranged. Some of the

Fig. 2.11. Electron micrograph showing mitochondria in a right ventricular myocyte of an adult guinea-pig. Note the closely packed cristae in regular array and the prominent matrix granules.

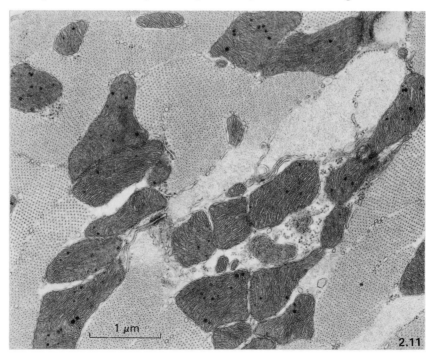

1 μm

2.11

mitochondria in myocardial cells are conspicuously large, occupying the length of four or more sarcomeres, and a few possess elongated tail-like extensions of the main organelle. They lie in closely packed columns which partially intersect the myofibrillar mass with which they come into close apposition and they are also closely apposed to T-tubules and lipid droplets where these are present.

The main functions of mitochondria are (1) the synthesis of ATP, and (2) calcium buffering, which is of particular interest in cardiac metabolism. The energy requirements for both these processes are provided by oxidative mitochondrial respiration, the substrates for which are derived from carbohydrates, lipids or proteins. In the absence of oxygen, as in total ischaemia, the production of ATP by oxidative phosphorylation is stopped and the only remaining source of ATP would be from glycolysis. Under such conditions, mitochondria become swollen and the intra-membrane particles become reduced first on the inner membrane but later on both inner and outer membranes (Ashraf, 1978); the swelling is initially reversible. However, even at maximum efficiency, glycolysis has been estimated to be capable of providing only about 20% of the ATP necessary for normal cell function (Opie, 1968). Contraction normally utilises about 75% of the total ATP production of the myocardial cell; so by stopping contraction during ischaemia or perfusion for transplant or for cardioplegia preparatory to surgical operation, the main energy drain is removed allowing the remaining ATP to be used to drive ionic pumps which are essential for the maintenance of cytoplasmic composition and cell volume. If the resumption of flow is quick enough, there could be a virtually complete recovery of normal cell function. The period of arrest can be prolonged by using hypothermic conditions which reduce the metabolic requirements even further (see Chapter 5).

Intracellular calcium concentration varies between approximately 10^{-7} and 10^{-5} M during relaxation and contraction respectively. There is now a considerable body of evidence that the mitochondria of cardiac myocytes may have a long-term buffering effect on the intracellular calcium concentration. Mitochondria are capable of accumulating calcium against a concentration gradient by way of respiration-dependent channels in the inner membrane and the release of Ca^{2+} from mitochondria appears to be effected by an independent mechanism. The calcium content of mitochondria is normally moderate but it is increased by contracture induced by caffeine (Wendt-Galitelli, Stöhr, Wolburg & Schlote, 1980). Possible models for the calcium influx and efflux systems are discussed by Williams (1983).

Mitochondrial ATPase has been localised in cardiac muscle by Ogawa & Mayohara (1969). It is situated on the inner membrane and its activity is considered to run in the direction of ATP synthesis, coupling oxidative metabolism to phosphorylation.

Other organelles

Microtubules, centrioles, microfilaments and leptofibrils

Microtubules have been described in cardiac myocytes (Sandborn, Côté, Roberge & Bois, 1967) but they are rather infrequent. When present, they lie either along the long axis of the myocyte parallel to the myofibrillae or transversely across the cell (Simpson, Rayns & Ledingham, 1973). Their functional role is unclear but by analogy with transport mechanisms in other cells, it is possible that they play a part in the rapid movement of atrial granules.

Centrioles composed of nine sets of triplet microtubules have been occasionally found in cardiac myocytes (Fawcett & McNutt, 1969) in sarcoplasmic cones adjacent to the nuclear poles. They are rather inconspicuous and tend to be missed on account of the crowded nature of these areas of the cell.

Microfilaments measuring 5–7 nm in diameter unassociated with thick filaments have been described by Sommer & Johnson (1979) in myocardial cells of the salamander and other species. Although they resemble actin filaments in other cells, it has not been established by immunocytochemical studies that these free-lying filaments are indeed composed of actin.

Leptofibrils are composed of small bundles of fine filaments about 5 nm in diameter showing a periodic banding by material resembling Z-lines. However, these lines occur at a periodicity of about 150 nm compared to 1.5–2.5 μm in myofibrillar complexes. They have been noted in the ventricular myocardium of several mammalian species but little is known of their chemical structure or of their possible function. Other unusual accumulations of filaments include the square lattice pattern found in the myocardium of ageing animals (Leeson, 1980; Feldman & Navaratnam, 1981; and see Chapter 7).

Metabolic storage organelles

The most conspicuous organelles associated with metabolic storage are glycogen granules which are freely present in the cytoplasm of most cardiac myocytes, and lipid droplets which are frequently found in ventricular myocytes but less commonly found in other cardiac cells. These organelles are described in further detail in Chapter 5.

Lysosomes, lipofuscin and peroxisomes

The formation of lipofuscin granules and the role played by lysosomes in this process are considered in Chapter 7. Peroxisomes are consistently present in cardiac myocytes; Hicks & Fahimi (1977) have drawn attention to their close spatial relationship to mitochondria, lipid droplets and junctional SR and have suggested a metabolic association between these organelles.

Atrial specific granules

The atrial myocardium in mammalian hearts is characterised by the presence of membrane-bound granules (Fig. 2.8) which are osmiophilic and contain peptides. The ultrastructural features of these granules and their possible physiological functions are discussed in Chapter 6.

———

The specialised ultrastructural features of cardiac myocytes mainly pertain to the cell membrane and cytoplasmic organelles and their prominence varies among different regions of the heart. Membrane apposition between myocytes includes specialised junctions such as nexuses, desmosomes and interfibrillar junctions and these may be grouped together to form intercalated discs which are complex and extensive in working myocardium and in the conducting bundle but not in specialised nodes. Sarcolemmal invaginations include T-tubules, which form an extensive network, and caveolae. The sarcoplasmic reticulum is extensive and parts of it form coupling arrangements with T-tubules and with the surface sarcolemma.

The myofibrillar mass is composed, as in skeletal muscle, of interdigitating thick filaments and thin filaments and the presence of Z-lines confers a similar sarcomeric pattern. The thick filaments are composed of myosin and the thin filaments are composed of actin associated with the regulatory proteins, tropomyosin and troponin. The chemical nature of these proteins in heart muscle may not be identical with that in skeletal muscle but the nature of contraction is likely to be similar. Mitochondria in cardiac myocytes occupy an unusually high proportion of cell volume and their cristae are closely packed in keeping with the enhanced functional demands related to oxidative respiration and calcium buffering; the mitochondria contain matrix granules which are probably associated with cytochrome oxidase activity. Other prominent features of cardiac myocytes include glycogen granules in enhanced quantity, lipid droplets, lipofuscin bodies and, in atrial myocardium, peptide-containing granules.

3

Nexuses (gap junctions) in heart muscle

Heart muscle functions physiologically as a syncytium and there is good evidence for the view that nexuses (also termed gap junctions or communicating junctions) constitute the structural basis for electrical coupling of adjacent cells (Dreifuss, Girardier & Forssmann, 1966; Weidmann, 1969; Hirakow & De Haan, 1970). The identification of nexuses as the relevant coupling sites is based on studies of excitable tissues but their presence in several other non-excitable tissues not known to exhibit coupling (Revel, Yee & Hudspeth, 1971; Loewenstein, 1981) indicates that they may serve other gating functions such as metabolic communication and transmission of signals during development. Such non-excitable tissues with nexuses include liver, lens, glial cells, epithelia and, as transitory features, numerous embryonic tissues. There have been occasional claims that electrical coupling of cells may be effected in the absence of any low-resistance membrane junctions (see Sperelakis & Mann, 1977) and that electrical interactions can be demonstrated across the extracellular space (Bennett & Spray, 1985) but there is little doubt that electronic coupling in the myocardium and other tissues, where it occurs, is dependent on nexuses. As far as we know, all nexuses in cardiac muscle are symmetrical there being no evidence of rectification either electrical or chemical. On the other hand, unidirectionally rectifying electronic junctions have been demonstrated in occasional sites such as the giant motor synapse of the crayfish (Giaume & Korn, 1985) and nexus permeability has been shown to be modifiable by chemical transmitters in the acinar cells of the pancreas in mammals and in retinal horizontal cells.

Assertions have been made in the past that nexuses are absent in the myocardium of avian and other non-mammalian hearts (Staley & Benson, 1966; Sommer & Johnson, 1969; Sperelakis, Meyer & MacDonald, 1970; Lemanski, Fitts & Marx, 1975) but such statements have been shown to be incorrect by more recent studies using thin sections and freeze-fracture replication (Martinez-Palomo & Mendez, 1971; Shibata & Yamamoto, 1979; Akester, 1981; Scheuermann & De Maziere, 1984). The latter studies have established that not only do nexuses occur in the myocardium of non-mammalian species but that they manifest several variations in arrangement. Thin-section studies of frog and fish myocardium have revealed punctate sites of very close membrane apposition (Kensler, Brink & Dewey, 1977; Santer, 1985); however, these sites are widely spaced and in freeze-fracture replicas they could correspond to nexus particles which are arranged in dispersed forms such as regular annuli surrounding particle-free areas of sarcolemma (Kensler *et al.*, 1977; Scheuermann & De Maziere, 1984). In other vertebrates, nexuses of variable length have been identified in thin sections and these correspond to macular aggregations of nexus particles in freeze-fracture replicas (Martinez-Palomo & Mendez, 1971; Martinez-Palomo & Alanis, 1980; Akester, 1981).

Detailed descriptions of the ultrastructural appearance of myocardial nexuses in thin sections and freeze-fracture replicas have been provided by numerous authors including Sjöstrand, Andersson-Cedergren & Dewey (1958), Dewey & Barr (1964), McNutt & Weinstein (1970), Simpson, Rayns & Ledingham (1973), McNutt (1975), Revel & Karnovsky (1967), Sommer & Johnson (1979), Page & Manjunath (1985) and Skepper & Navaratnam (1986). Moreover, much has been learned about their chemical composition and likely mechanism of action by X-ray diffraction, biochemical analysis and immunochemical studies.

Ultrastructural appearances of nexuses

A nexus is formed by the close apposition of the plasmalemma of two abutting cells and, though it was originally believed that the outer leaflets of the apposing membranes are fused to form a pentalaminar structure which occludes the intercellular space, Revel & Karnovsky (1967) established the existence of a distinct though labyrinthine gap, 2 nm wide, which can be demonstrated by an extracellular tracer such as colloidal lanthanum hydroxide or horseradish peroxidase. True tight junctons where the intercellular space is occluded by outer leaflet fusion are not found in definitive heart muscle although they are present in other tissues especially in epithelia, including the myocardial epithelium of early mammalian embryos (see Chapter 1).

In general, a correlation can be made between the size of cells and the size of nexuses joining them. The smaller the cell, the more difficult it is to find nexuses, some of which are restricted to punctate appositions. This is so of early embryonic heart cells, of definitive myocardial cells in lower vertebrates and of nodal cells in mammals. The correlation is in keeping with the expected differences in input resistance; the larger the cell, the lower the input resistance and hence the lower the coupling resistance required. Nonetheless, nexuses in the working myocardium are still relatively small in comparison to the length of myocytes; the lengths of membrane apposition in the rat are commonly in the 0.5–1 μm range though some may extend for up to 3 μm. They are usually oriented parallel to the long axis of the myocyte, forming all or part of a longitudinal step within an intercalated disc, or elsewhere along the sides of the fibre.

The nexus is usually flanked on one or both cytoplasmic sides by relatively clear areas free of particles and organelles. Nevertheless, in heart muscle and in neural tissue, some non-fibrillar fuzzy material is seen closely attached to the cytoplasmic face of each membrane (Sommer & Johnson, 1979; Page & Manjunath, 1986) a feature which is absent in liver gap junctions. Recently it has been shown that this fuzzy layer, which seems to be a feature of gap junctions in excitable tissues but not in others, can be removed by exposure to trypsin or proteolysis by serine protease; it is thought to be composed of a subunit of molecular weight 14 500–17 500 daltons covalently linked to the main nexus channel protein (see below) which lies in the lipid bilayer of the plasmalemma.

Tangential sections through nexuses reveal a hexagonal lattice with an approximately 10-nm spacing and, in preparations that are exposed to heavy metal stains such as osmium, the hexagons exhibit an electron-dense centre. Preparations in which the extracellular space has been delineated by colloidal lanthanum demonstrate that the hexagons comprise columns or bridges connecting the two cell membranes across the 2-nm gap.

The concept that bridges extend across the intercellular gap has been strengthened by numerous freeze-fracture studies on various tissues especially heart and liver. These studies show that there is a hexagonal array of particles with a centre-to-centre spacing of 7–11 nm on the P face, i.e. on the intramembranous aspect of the inner (cytoplasmic) leaflet of the plasmalemma, and there is a similar hexagonal array of pits on the E face, i.e. on the intramembranous aspect of the outer leaflet. Particle size lies in the 7–11-nm range but, when a goniometer stage with a rotating specimen holder is used to reduce tilt errors accompanied by measurement of particle diameter at a specific orientation to the direction of shadowing, the measurements lie at the upper end of the range (Kensler, Brink & Dewey, 1977; Skepper & Navaratnam, 1986). The general belief is that the particles on the P face are in register with the pits on the E face, a view which is supported by detailed analysis of complementary replicas of both fracture faces, but Page & Manjunath (1985) have recently questioned this interpretation. Be that as it may, nexus particles have been confirmed to contain channels which connect the cytoplasmic compartments of the two abutting cells. When the shadowing is favourable, the P-face particles occasionally display a central depression which some authors have interpreted as representing the central hydrophilic channel; the electron-dense centre in the hexagons revealed by tangential thin sections is probably a similar manifestation. The particles in each membrane have been estimated, by correlating shadow length with angle of shadowing, to be about 7.5 nm in height (at right angles to the membrane surface) so that when the membranes are suitably apposed with particles in alignment, the enclosed channel measures about 15 nm which is compatible with the distance between the two cytoplasmic compartments.

X-ray diffraction studies correlated with analysis of electron micrographs have inferred that each particle is composed of six subunits enclosing a hydrophilic core (Caspar *et al.*, 1977; Makowski *et al.*, 1977). Fourier analysis of electron-microscopic views at different tilts have confirmed the presence of six subunits, each measuring 2.5 nm in diameter and 7.5 nm in height, and of a central channel 2 nm at the intercellular end but which narrows slightly within the membrane (Unwin & Zampighi, 1980). These authors also described a second population of particle with a smaller aperture which they interpreted as the closed state of the channel. They proposed a model for the configuration of a particle whereby rotation of the subunits would close the hydrophilic channel.

The passage of not only small ions but also large hydrophilic molecules from cell to cell was demonstrated by Kanno & Loewenstein (1964) when they found that fluorescein (330 daltons) traverses the junctional pathway. This was shown initially in cells carrying electrical signals but subsequently also in epithelia and glia. Three fundamental properties of the junctional pathway were enunciated by Loewenstein and his colleagues: (i) High flux rates for hydrophilic molecules. (ii) Moderate molecular size limit (the range appears to be 200–2500 daltons dependent on species and tissue; vertebrate junctions appear to be restricted to the lower end of the range, probably less than 500 daltons). And (iii) the pathway is leakproof to the exterior and hence is electrically well insulated from the main extracellular space.

Chemical composition of nexus particles (connexons)

There is as yet no general agreement on the precise molecular configuration of the major nexus protein which has been given the term connexin (Goodenough, 1975). Chemical studies of membrane fractions rich in nexuses showed at most a few non-glycosylated protein species. In rat and mouse liver, Hertzberg & Gilula (1979) and Henderson, Eibl & Weber (1979) found a major species of molecular weight 26–27 kD which fits in with the dimension of nexus subunits. Many investigators believe that the principal component in most animal species is a 25–28-kD protein (Hertzberg & Skibbens, 1984) but reported sizes range from 10 to 54 kD. Many of these differences could be caused by degradation or aggregation of the nexus protein or by the presence of precursor molecules but the biochemical relationship between the various proteins has not yet been clarified.

Early studies of cell communication in heterologous co-culture led to the notion that nexuses in different tissues might be composed of highly homologous polypeptides (Michalke & Loewenstein, 1971; Epstein & Gilula, 1977). However, subsequent analyses of nexuses isolated from the heart, liver and lens indicated differences in polypeptide composition (Hertzberg et al., 1982; Gros, Nicholson & Revel, 1983; Nicholson et al., 1983). Using sheep antibody raised to rat liver nexus protein, Hertzberg & Skibbens (1984) tested its cross-reactivity against several other tissues and found a 27-kD polypeptide that binds the antibodies in liver, pancreas, heart, brain, stomach, kidney, adrenal gland, ovary and uterus; only lens fibre cells failed to cross-react. In similar tests for species specificity of nexus polypeptide, these authors found binding of antibody to 27-kD polypeptides in the livers of representatives of all vertebrate classes, which was strongest in mammals, but no cross-reaction was observed in invertebrate tissues.

Dermietzel et al. (1984) reported somewhat different results when testing the cross-reactivity of rabbit antiserum raised against mouse liver 26-kD protein. Strong reaction was observed in the liver, exocrine pancreas, kidney, small intestine, fallopian tube, endometrium and myometrium whereas only weak fluorescence was found in the endocrine pancreas and none in the myocardium, ovaries and lens. These results taken together with those of Hertzberg & Skibbens (1984; see also Hertzberg & Spray, 1985) suggest that, whereas liver and myocardial nexuses may share antigenic sites that can be recognised by certain antibodies, there are other antigenic sites in liver which are absent or inaccessible in heart muscle. Peptide mapping has revealed differences in amino acid sequences in the major nexus polypeptide in different tissues, e.g. in the liver and heart (Gros, Nicholson & Revel, 1983). Moreover, Warner & Lawrence (1982) and Blennerhassett & Caveney (1983) have suggested that there are functional differences, with possibly underlying structural differences, between nexuses even in the same tissue. Nevertheless, although there are variations in nexus protein structure in different species and different tissues, and possibly in the same tissue, there is evidence that the differences are masked to some extent by folding of the molecule which yields a more homologous final structure.

Variations in nexus structure within the myocardium

Williams & De Haan (1981) considered the feasibility of defining a minimal functional nexus as an aggregation of four channels which need not be arranged in any particular pattern. However, they found that, in certain circumstances, nexus particles need not be aggregated at all for electrical coupling which can be effected by isolated channels spread over a relatively wide area of membrane apposition. In *Xenopus* myocardium, the only nexuses reported have been linear strands of particles (Mazet, 1977). Similar strands and other variations have been observed in mammals, fairly commonly in the embryonic myocardium (Gros, Mocquard, Challice & Schrevel, 1978; Navaratnam *et al.*, 1986b) and more rarely in adults (Shibata, Nakata & Page, 1980; Skepper, Thurley & Navaratnam, 1982). If nexuses do comprise sites of electrical coupling in heart muscle, one might expect them to be less evident in regions of slow impulse conduction such as the atrioventricular node and, in fact, some investigators have reported them to be sparse or even absent in the nodes of certain mammalian species (De Fellice & Challice, 1969; Hayashi, 1971; Virágh & Porte, 1973; Mochet, Moravec, Guillemot & Hatt, 1975).

The ultrastructure of nexuses in the atrioventricular node of young adult (4–8 months) female golden hamsters was studied in the author's laboratory, using thin sections and freeze-fracture replicas, and compared with that of nexuses in the working myocardium of the right ventricular wall (Skepper & Navaratnam, 1986). Care was taken to orientate the surface plane of the replica at 90° to the incident electron beam when micrographs were being prepared so as to minimise tilt errors in measurement. The magnification was calibrated by using a line grating of $2160\,mm^{-1}$. Measurements of nexus particle diameter were taken, at 90° to the direction of shadowing, from prints at × 90 000 using an eyepiece graticule in a Wild M 50 microscope operated at × 12.

Measurements of annular and macular nexus particles were made from at least five hearts in each instance. Each junction was taken as one sample and n represents the total number of junctions examined (Table 3.1). This allows for variations between junctions, between replicas and between animals. Where appropriate, measurements of particles in annular and macular nexuses were compared using Student's t-test.

Table 3.1 *Measurements of annular nexuses from atrioventricular node (AVN) myocytes and of macular nexuses from right ventricular (RV) myocardium after freeze-fracture replication*

	Annular nexus (AVN) Mean ± s.e.m. (n) Total measurements	Macular nexus (RV) Mean ± s.e.m. (n) Total measurements
	nm	nm
Particle diameter	10.59 ± 0.07 (43) 993	10.95 ± 0.04 (25) 788
Central depression diameter	1.7 to 2.5	1.7 to 2.5
Centre-to-centre spacing	10.83 ± 0.09 (10) 310	10.99 ± 0.045 (5) 256
Particle-free area diameter	59.4 ± 0.46 (36) 325	
Central particle diameter	12.04 ± 0.26 (12) 12	

Figures in parentheses indicate the numbers of nexuses sampled.

Nexuses in the right ventricular myocardium of the hamster

In the right ventricular wall, nexuses are encountered only at the site of intercalated discs and, within the discs, they are predominantly restricted to areas of sarcolemma oriented parallel to the long axis of contiguous myocytes. This orientation is seen in thin sections and also in freeze-fracture replicas (Figs. 3.1, 3.2). The form of nexus is uniformly of the macular type with a surrounding particle-sparse zone of sarcolemma (Fig. 3.2). The maculae comprise closely packed arrays of particles of the P face of the fractured sarcolemma, the particles having a mean diameter of 10.95 ± 0.04 nm (s.e.m.) (Fig. 3.3 and Table 3.1) with a range of 9.5 to 12.4 nm. Where the direction of shadowing is favourable, it is possible to see a central depression, about 1.7–2.5 nm in diameter, on the particle (inset Fig. 3.2). The mean centre-to-centre spacing of particles on the P face is 10.99 ± 0.045 nm (Table 3.1).

Nexuses in the atrioventricular node of the hamster

Nodal myocytes are recognised by their narrow diameter, paucity of T-tubule invaginations and relative profusion of caveolae. Very few typical intercalated discs are found in thin sections; instead, junctional contacts between adjacent myocytes are short and they occur most frequently at the lateral cell surface. Nexuses are sparse and are either punctate (Fig. 3.4) or of very short length. In freeze-fracture replicas of nodal material, several varieties of nexus are

Fig. 3.1. Thin section of right ventricular myocardium of a golden hamster showing an extensive intercalated disc which includes several nexuses (N), desmosomes (D) and intermediate junctions (I).

Fig. 3.2. Freeze-fracture replica of right ventricular myocardium showing an extensive intercalated disc which includes a macular nexus on a longitudinally orientated part of the disc. The plane of cleavage has exposed the 'P' and 'E' faces of the apposing membranes. Arrow in circle indicates the direction of shadowing. The inset at the top left-hand corner shows an enlargement ($\times$ 300 000) of nexus particles some of which possess a distinct central depression.

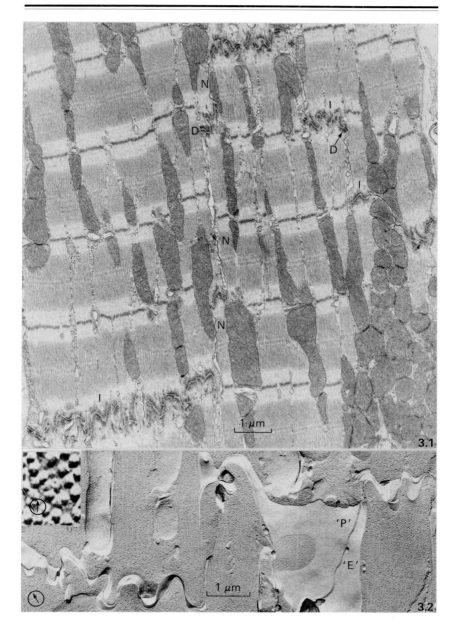

observed (Figs. 3.5, 3.6), mostly on the lateral aspect of myocytes. They include maculae but these are few in number and generally smaller in size than nexuses in the right ventricular myocardium, some containing fewer than fifteen particles (Fig. 3.5). Short linear strands of particles are also found (Fig. 3.5) but annular nexuses are

Fig. 3.3. Histograms showing the normal distribution of particle diameter measurements: (A) in macular nexuses of the right ventricular myocardium; and (B) in the annular nexuses of the atrioventricular node.

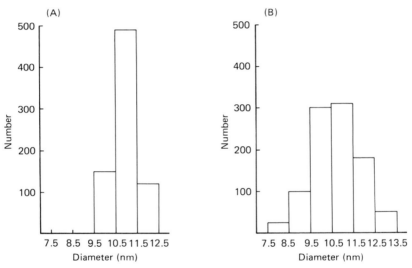

Fig. 3.4. Thin section of atrioventricular node region showing cell junctions including desmosomes (D), punctate nexuses (arrows) and a length of nexus apposition (N).

Fig. 3.5. Freeze-fracture replica of atrioventricular node showing a variety of forms of nexus, including a small macular nexus (A), a macular nexus attached to a curved row of particles (B), an annular nexus with some infilling (C), and a short line of particles (D).

Fig. 3.6. Freeze-fracture replica showing an annular nexus in the atrioventricular node region. There are central depressions in some of the annular nexus particles (double-headed arrows). Note also the presence of isolated large particles (single-headed arrow) in the particle-sparse zone just outside the nexus.

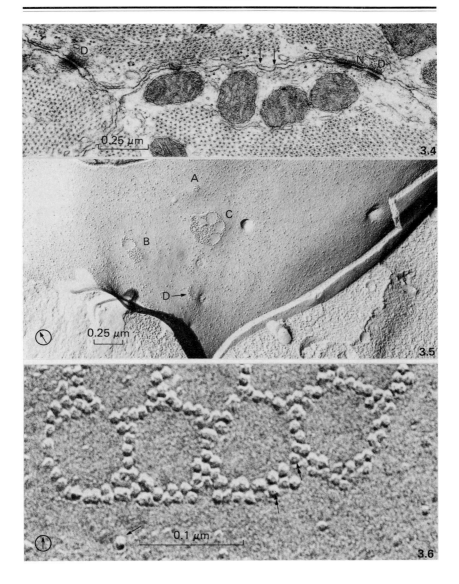

the commonest variety present in the node; Fig. 3.7 shows a typical annular nexus situated where the extracellular space is narrowed and comprising regular, linked annuli of particles surrounding particle-free areas of membrane.

The particles have a mean diameter of 10.59 ± 0.07 nm (Fig. 3.3 and Table 3.1) with a mean centre-to-centre spacing of 10.83 ± 0.09 nm. When these figures are compared with those for molecular nexuses in the right ventricle using Student's t-test there is no significant difference in the centre-to-centre spacings but there is a significant difference ($P<0.001$) between the diameters of the particles in the two types of nexus. Where the shadowing is favourable (Fig. 3.6), it is possible to see a central depression (1.7–2.5 nm in diameter) on some particles of the annular nexus similar to depressions seen in macular nexuses of the right ventricular myocardium. The particle-free areas of the annuli are circular in profile with a mean diameter of 59.4 ± 0.46 nm (Table 3.1).

The number of annuli in a single nexus ranges from one to as many as fifty and, occasionally, a single large particle (mean diameter 12.04 nm) is seen in the centre of the otherwise particle-free area enclosed by the annulus (Fig. 3.7). The area immediately surrounding the entire annular nexus group contains fewer particles than the general sarcolemma but, occasionally, a few particles of similar diameter to larger nexus particles and with similar central depressions are found scattered in this particle-sparse zone (Figs. 3.6, 3.8).

Variations in the pattern of aggregation of particles in annular nexuses are observed. Linear strands or 'arms' of particles linked to annuli are frequently seen (Fig. 3.8) and various degrees of filling within annuli are also present. These range from a loose accumulation of particles equivalent in area to one or more annuli, located centrally or peripherally or in both regions, of an otherwise annular nexus (Figs. 3.5, 3.8). Generally, nexuses composed of the largest number of linked annuli (10 or more) are composed entirely of open annuli.

The foregoing ultrastructural observations on the hamster heart indicate that the general myocardium, represented by the right ventricle, contains macular type nexuses only while myocytes in the atrioventricular node display punctate, linear and annular forms in addition to small maculae. Moreover, there is a small but significant difference in nexus particle diameter between the two regions.

Measurements of nexus particle diameter have been commonly cited as 6–8 nm for vertebrate nexuses in general (Loewenstein, 1981) and 7–10 nm for myocardial nexuses in particular (McNutt & Weinstein, 1970). The present figures of 10.59 nm and 10.95 nm for nodal and right ventricular myocardium respectively of the hamster are both significantly higher. This is probably due to the use of a goniometer stage with rotating specimen holder to minimise tilt errors (Willison & Rowe, 1980; Navaratnam, Thurley

Fig. 3.7. Freeze-fracture replica of the atrioventricular node region showing a large nexus with numerous annuli exposed on the E face of a cell membrane.

Fig. 3.8. Freeze-fracture replica of the atrioventricular node region showing (A) a nexus comprising a single annulus linked to a short, curved row of particles (note the presence of a few large isolated particles, indicated by arrows, in the particle-sparse zone surrounding the nexus) and (B) an annular nexus with a degree of infilling. In B, both P and E faces have been exposed.

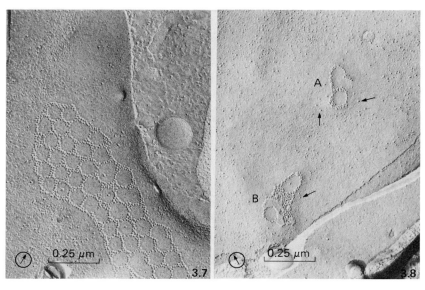

& Skepper, 1982), and also to measuring particle diameters at a specific orientation in respect to the direction of shadow casting. Kensler, Brink & Dewey (1977) also took care to standardise their measurements of ventricular annular nexus particles in the frog and their mean figure of 10.4 nm is close to the present observations. A third possible reason for high values for a particle diameter is the capping effect of unidirectional shadowing (Willison & Rowe, 1980). It is possible that our quartz monitor, while confirming that similar thicknesses of metal were being deposited (as shown by small intersample variations reflected by low S.E.M. values), was not calibrated in absolute terms and could have read uniformly low values. However, the low intersample variation and the precise nature of the conditions under which the replicas were produced and examined render it valid to compare measurements from different regions of the heart. Dahl & Isenberg (1980) and Shibata & Page (1981) have suggested that low *intracellular* calcium levels could cause an increase in nexus particle size but we have not found differences in particle size between animals perfused with saline with or without calcium.

The small discrepancy in diameter between particles in the right ventricle and in the atrioventricular node could be explained by (i) an intrinsic difference in protein molecular size at the two sites or (ii) by a functional difference such as different ratios of open to closed channels or (iii) by conformational changes in the particles caused by differences in packing. The first possibility, though unlikely, cannot be ruled out in view of the queries raised by Warner & Lawrence (1982) and Blennerhassett & Caveney (1983) about the uniformity of nexuses even within the same tissue. The second possibility seems unlikely because of the normal distribution of particle size measurements in each region (Fig. 3.3). Dahl & Isenberg (1980) used freeze-fracture replication to demonstrate that nexus particles on sheep Purkinje cells usually have a mean diameter of 8.3 nm with a range of 7–10 nm and their histograms revealed a normal distribution with a single modal value. On the other hand, when the Purkinje cells were treated with the uncoupling agent dinitrophenol, a second population of particles with a mean diameter of 10.8 nm appeared giving the histograms a bimodal distribution. In the present study, measurements of ventricular and nodal nexal particles both show normal distribution each with a single modal value (Fig. 3.3) suggesting that the difference in mean diameter is unlikely to be due to a difference in the ratio of coupled to uncoupled channels. Peracchia & Girsch (1985) have argued that there are three forces which help to maintain particle packing within nexuses, (a) a binding force between opposite particles on apposing cell membranes, (b) a repulsive force between neighbouring particles, and (c) a repulsive force between peri-junctional membrane surfaces. It seems likely that the small difference in particle diameters between macular and annular nexuses is caused by variations in the repulsive force between neighbouring particles reflecting differences in packing arrangement in the two types of nexus. Peracchia & Girsch also suggested that the packing arrangement could be maintained by filamentous bridges between particles but we have not been able to confirm the presence of such bridges in our fractured material.

Central depressions, similar to those observed by McNutt & Weinstein (1970), were seen in the present study in a proportion of junction particles of annular nexuses as well as of maculae. The depression measured 1.7–2.5 nm in diameter which correlates well with the dimensions of the hydrophilic pore in nexus particles estimated by the use of fluorescent probes (Loewenstein, 1981). The presence of characteristic central depressions in particles arranged in annular form provides circumstantial evidence that they constitute true nexuses and the fact that the appearances of the P and E faces at the same nexus match each other confirms that these particles do bridge the gap between the apposed membranes.

Aggregation and removal of nexuses

Details of the process by which nexus particles aggregate are unclear and hence there is little understanding why nexuses are arranged in different forms. There is evidence to indicate that nexus protein (connexin) is synthesised in the cytoplasm (Loewenstein, 1981) and that it is then inserted into the plasmalemma forming a pool of particles which subsequently aggregate to form nexuses. The observation of occasional isolated nexus particles, characterised by typical diameter and central depression, within the otherwise particle-free zone surrounding annular or macular nexuses supports this hypothesis. It is also probable that the plasma membrane contains large amounts of morphologically unrecognisable nexus precursors because nexuses have been shown to assemble rapidly even in the absence of ATP or protein synthesis.

A possible sequence is that particles accumulate at specific sites, or formation plaques, in the plasmalemma orientating themselves into groups, with occasional linear strands, and then pack to form a macular nexus. As the particles move into the group, a particle-sparse zone becomes apparent round the growing nexus (Friend & Gilula, 1972; Albertini & Anderson, 1974; Gros et al., 1978; Yee & Revel, 1978). However, later stages of enlargement of nexuses are said to be associated with the appearance of particle-free aisles within the nexus which are subsequently filled by new particles (Albertini & Anderson, 1974; Decker & Friend, 1974; Albertini, Fawcett & Olds, 1975; Decker, 1976; Elias & Friend, 1976; Kogon & Pappas, 1976; Shibata, Nakata & Page, 1980).

Two processes have been suggested for the removal of nexuses. They may be internalised (Larsen, 1983; Mazet, Wittenberg & Spray, 1985) or lateral particle dispersion may occur causing the appearance of large, central particle-free aisles (Lane & Swales, 1980; Lee, Cran & Lane, 1982). Cytoplasmic vesicles have been observed frequently near the nexus segments of intercalated discs in the myocardium (Figs. 3.9, 3.10), supporting the view that nexuses can be degraded by internalisation. Larsen and his colleagues have studied similar vesicles in the granulosa cells of the rabbit ovary and have concluded that nexuses are endocytosed by an actin-dependent mechanism. It is not clear what the ultimate fate of these endocytosed functional elements may be. Are they degraded completely by the lysosomal system or are the junctional proteins recycled and utilised again by the plasma membrane? If nexuses are deleted and rapidly reassembled, as they appear to be in regenerating liver, the process is more likely to depend on lateral dispersal and recongregation than on internalisation and recombination. One would expect that internalisation and fusion with lysosomes would inflict irreversible loss of function.

Annular nexuses

The presence of annular nexuses presents a further enigma. Our results clearly demonstrate that punctate, linear, annular and macular nexuses of different sizes co-exist in the atrioventricular node of the hamster. There is evidence in some species that either the linear or the annular form could comprise the sole type of nexus between electronically coupled cardiac myocytes (Mazet & Cartaud, 1976; Kensler *et al.*, 1977; Mazet, 1977) and in culture it has been demonstrated that isolated or dispersed protochannels are sufficient for electronic communication (Williams & De Haan,

Fig. 3.9. Thin section of left atrial myocardium of an 18-month-old rat showing the nexus component of an intercalated disc with part of the nexus internalised to form a vesicle-like profile.

Fig. 3.10. Thin section of left atrial myocardium of a 21-month-old rat showing part of a nexus internalised to form a vesicle-like profile.

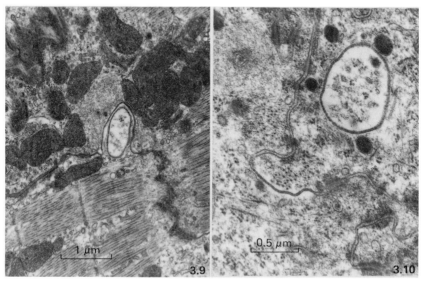

1981). This would suggest that all varieties of nexus are capable of forming communicating channels given the appropriate stimulus but the reason for their co-existence in a particular tissue remains obscure. The partial infilling of some annular nexuses suggests that they could be an intermediate stage in the formation of maculae. Such infilling was usually found in nexuses with relatively few annuli and only once encountered where there were more than ten annuli in the junction. This adds further weight to the hypothesis that variations in nexus pattern such as annuli are competent coupling junctions in their own right.

The uniform diameter of the particle-free areas enclosed in annular junctions is difficult to explain. Recent studies employing cholesterol probes on frog myocardium (Mazet, 1985) suggest that the biochemical composition of the membrane enclosed within the annuli is different from that of the sarcolemma outside. The manner in which this difference is generated is not clear, nor is it known whether the special chemical nature of this area could explain how protochannel particles accumulate. In an earlier study on cultured hepatocytes, Robinek, Jung & Gebhard (1982) suggested that the enclosed areas constitute formation zones for macular nexuses. It is possible to speculate that these areas represent sites of fusion of intracellular membranous vesicles to produce nexus formation plaques but much more evidence is required to substantiate such a hypothesis.

A considerable range of nexus patterns in myocardial and other tissues have been described in the literature (Martinez-Palomo & Mendez, 1971; Raviola & Gilula, 1973; Pricam, Humbert, Perrelet & Orci, 1974; Kensler et al., 1977; Mazet, 1977; Mazet & Cartaud, 1977; Gros et al., 1978; Shibata & Yamamoto, 1979; Shibata et al., 1980; Akester, 1981; Williams & De Haan, 1981; Navaratnam et al., 1986; Scheuermann & De Maziere, 1984) so it would appear that the packing arrangement of particles is secondary to their function as transcellular channels or it may vary according to the requirements of the relevant cells.

Variations in nexus morphology in the hamster heart which have been described in the present study may reflect the different roles played by the nodal myocytes and the working myocardium. One should not lose sight of the fact that the hamster is a hibernating species, capable of pronounced bradycardia, and the predominance of annular nexuses in the atrioventricular node may be related to this feature. Further investigations, especially in regard to the molecular structure of different nexus types, are necessary before it becomes possible to explain their precise roles in the functions of general myocardium and of the specialised nodal and conducting tissues in the heart.

———

At nexuses, the gap between the apposed cell membranes measures about 2 nm and it is bridged by hexameric particles on each membrane abutting similar particles across the gap. Each particle contains a narrow hydrophilic channel and the alignment permits restricted communication between the cytoplasmic compartments of the coupled cells. The principal component of nexus particles in most animal species is likely to be a 25–28-kD protein. Immunochemical studies suggest that the protein, though similar, is not necessarily identical in different species nor in different organs of the same species.

The pattern of nexus particle arrangement may show variation even within the same organ. In the golden hamster heart, there is evidence of such variation especially between working myocardium and nodal myocardium. In the musculature of the right ventricle the particles are grouped to give the appearance of maculae in freeze-fracture preparations and that of fairly long segments of membrane apposition in thin-section electron micrographs. Such nexuses usually occupy part of a longitudinal step of an intercalated disc and they are characterised by the presence of fuzzy material on the cytoplasmic surface of each membrane. In the AV node, on the other hand, nexuses are sparse and either punctate or of very short length in thin sections. In freeze-fracture replicas they may take the form of small patches, linear configurations or, most commonly, of annuli of particles surrounding a particle-free area. Measurements made on electron micrographs, after allowing for tilt of the specimen, yielded a small but significant difference in nexus particle diameter in the right ventricle (10.95 nm) compared with the AV node (10.59 nm) which is likely to be caused by dissimilarities in packing.

4

T-tubules and couplings with sarcoplasmic reticulum

Transversely orientated tubules invaginated from the sarcolemma were described in myocardial cells as early as 1957 by Lindner who observed them in the ventricular musculature of the dog. However, the possible significance of these invaginations was not appreciated until similar tubules, which came to be known as T-tubules, were seen in skeletal muscle cells and were implicated in excitation–contraction coupling (for reviews see Endo, 1977; Fabiato, 1977). Since then the extent and nature of the T-system in mammalian myocardial cells has been studied by many investigators including Simpson & Oertalis (1961, 1962), Nelson & Benson (1963), Simpson (1965), Page (1967a,b,1968), Rayns, Simpson & Bertaud (1968), Fawcett & McNutt (1969), Hibbs & Ferrans (1969), Forssmann & Girardier (1970), Naylor & Merrillees (1971), Forbes & Sperelakis (1977), Ayettey & Navaratnam (1978a, 1980), Forbes, Hawkey & Sperelakis (1984) and Navaratnam et al. (1986a). Cytochemical studies show that T-tubule membrane resembles the surface sarcolemma in the localisation of adenylate and guanylate cyclases (Schultze, 1984) and of basic ATPase (Malouf & Meissner, 1984).

Among vertebrate hearts a T-system has been described only in mammals although its presence has been reported in some invertebrate species. It is now generally recognised that, in typical ventricular myocytes of mammals, tubular invaginations of the sarcolemma recur more or less periodically at or near the Z-lines where they are frequently coupled with elements of the sarcoplasmic reticulum (SR). Such primary T-tubules are usually substantial in size and they characteristically possess a luminal coating of basement membrane. In most species, including rat and dog and man, they have a mean diameter of 100–150 nm; however, in a seemingly unrelated set of species which includes hamsters, bats and seals, the primary T-tubules are exceptionally large ranging from 350 to 500 nm in diameter.

Early investigators had difficulty in determining the full extent of the T-system and they regarded all longitudinally orientated tubules as part of the SR because neither a connection to the sarcolemma nor a coating of basement membrane could be discerned. In recent years, however, infiltration techniques using tracers such as ferritin, lanthanum salts, horseradish peroxidase or osmium-potassium ferrocyanide have demonstrated that the T-system comprises more than transverse invaginations at Z-line level. For instance, systematic studies of the rat myocardium after peroxidase labelling show that several branches arise from the primary invaginations and course in different planes (Forssmann & Girardier, 1970; Ayettey & Navaratnam, 1978a). These branches are generally narrower than the parent tubules but the presence of peroxidase enables them to be assigned as part of the T-system, rather than the SR, which is coupled not only to the primary T-tubules but also to the narrower ramifying branches including longitudinal elements. In addition, it has long been known that, like smooth muscle but unlike most skeletal muscle, cardiac muscle exhibits similar extensive couplings between the surface sarcolemma and superficial SR cisterns (Page, 1968) and these are frequently seen near intercalated discs.

When the various reports in the literature are compared, it appears that the degree of differentiation of the T-system depends on the region of the heart. For instance, Forssmann & Girardier (1970) reported that whereas a T-system is present in all of the ventricular myocardium, it is found only in a fraction of atrial cells in the rat. Moreover, there is much support for the view that T-tubules are poorly developed or absent in the specialised nodal and conducting systems (see Ayettey & Navaratnam, 1978a, for references). The present chapter comprises a systematic study, employing labelling with horseradish peroxidase, of the distribution and character of T-tubules in different parts of the rat heart including the general ventricular and atrial myocardium and representative regions of the specialised nodal and conducting systems. The pattern in the rat will then be compared with that in the golden hamster where the T-tubules are considerably larger.

Rat myocardium

Adult albino rats of the CFHB strain were used for horseradish peroxidase infiltration of heart muscle in which 3,3′-diaminobenzidine was used as chromogen (see Ayettey & Navaratnam, 1978a, for details of technique). The material was then osmicated, dehydrated and embedded before thin sections were cut for transmission electron microscopy. This material was complemented by representative freeze-fracture preparations which provide a contrasting view of T-tubules.

General ventricular myocardium

In typical ventricular myocardial cells it is possible to discern several components of the T-system, namely (a) primary transverse tubules, (b) secondary transverse tubules, (c) longitudinal tubules, and (d) tertiary tubules.

(a) Primary transverse tubules are direct invaginations of the sarcolemma (Fig. 4.1) which are orientated at right angles to the long axis of the myocyte; they measure about 130 nm in diameter and penetrate deep into the cytoplasm to end near the I-bands of the myofibrillae (Figs. 4.1, 4.2, 4.3, 4.4). In freeze-fracture replicas, their openings are regularly arranged and can be distinguished from the mouths of caveolae which are smaller, more numerous and dispersed in irregular fashion (see Fig. 2.1); in some preparations where the plane of cleavage is suitable, it is possible to study the particle pattern on T-tubule membranes; the particles are dispersed irregularly on the P face with a density of about $200\,\mu m^{-2}$. There are numerous sites at which cisterns of SR are closely apposed or coupled to primary invaginations (Figs. 4.1, 4.3, 4.4).

(b) Secondary T-tubules arise directly from the primary invaginations (Fig. 4.3) and run across the long axis of the cell at about the level of the I-band and Z-line; they are fairly narrow (50 nm diameter) and do not appear to give off any branches. Typical couplings occur between the secondary T-tubules and adjacent profiles of SR, but they are less frequent than couplings in relation to primary tubules.

(c) Longitudinal tubules of the T-system are also direct branches of the primary invaginations; they run parallel to the myofibrillae (Figs. 4.2, 4.5) and many can be followed over the entire length of a sarcomere but there is no evidence to suggest that any of these longitudinal tubules transgress Z-lines. Longitudinal tubules are narrower than the parent transverse tubules, usually measuring about 64 nm in diameter. Typical couplings with adjacent SR profiles can be observed.

(d) Tertiary transverse tubules are very narrow (25–30 nm in diameter) channels occasionally found linking adjacent longitudinal tubules at the A-band level of the myofibrillae; within the A-band they are absent from the H-zone, i.e. they occur where the thick filaments are overlapped by thin filaments. Couplings between these elements and the SR have been observed in many preparations.

The sarcoplasmic reticulum (SR) in ventricular myocardial cells comprises a system of channels widely ramified in the cytoplasm (Fig. 4.1). These SR channels are narrower (about 38 nm in

Fig. 4.1. Electron micrograph of left ventricular myocardium of young adult rat (6 months) showing a series of primary T-tubules, at Z-line or I-band level, most of which are coupled with cisterns of junctional sarcoplasmic reticulum (SR). Note the luminal lining of basement membrane in the T-tubules.

Fig. 4.2. Left ventricular myocardium of young adult rat labelled with horseradish peroxidase to show the extent of the T-system. Primary and secondary transverse tubules as well as longitudinal branches are found.

Fig. 4.3. Left ventricular myocardium of young adult rat labelled with horseradish peroxidase. Note secondary transverse branches (T_2) and longitudinal branches (T_L) and SR couplings.

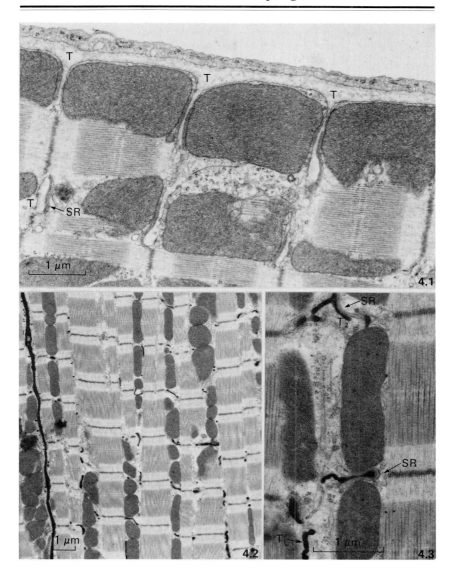

Fig. 4.4. Freeze-fracture replica of rat left ventricular myocardium showing T-tubules and SR cisterns. Arrow in circle indicates the direction of shadowing.

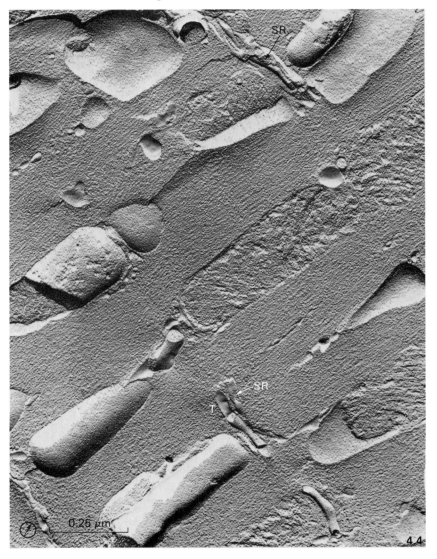

diameter) than any part of the T-system except the tertiary T-tubules. Most of the SR forms an interconnecting system more-or-less investing the myofibrillae throughout their length, there being continuity in the system by way of narrow isthmus-like connections across Z-line level. Impressive three-dimensional perspectives of the SR network can be obtained by employing high-voltage electron microscopy of thick sections (Peachey, Waugh & Sommer, 1974).

As emphasised earlier, the SR forms numerous couplings with the T-system, especially in relation to primary tubules, and with the surface sarcolemma (Fig. 4.6). The profiles of SR which are so coupled are characterised by the presence of intraluminal granules and cone-shaped electron-dense processes which extend from the SR across the cytoplasmic gap (10–12 nm wide) towards, but not touching, the invaginated or surface sarcolemmal membrane. Unlike the appearance in skeletal myocytes, the SR cisterns related to primary T-tubules cannot be accurately termed terminal sacs since they often curve over the apposed T-tubule to continue from one sarcomeric region to the next and, moreover, they are not dilated compared with other parts of the SR (*free* SR; mean diameter 38 nm). In other words, these cisterns in heart muscle tend to be intercalated into the free SR, unlike in skeletal muscle where they form terminal cul-de-sacs. For these reasons, the term *junctional SR* is preferred to cover these cisterns which are closely apposed to T-tubules or surface sarcolemma and have the characteristic features of intraluminal granules and junctional processes (Sommer & Johnson, 1979); it has been estimated that junctional SR accounts for about 20% of total SR. Occasionally, SR cisterns equipped with membrane processes and intraluminal granules have been reported in positions apparently unrelated to T-tubules or surface sarcolemma and Sommer & Johnson have proposed the term *extended junctional SR* to describe these profiles. A similarly puzzling feature is that cisterns identical in appearance to junctional SR have been described near the Z-line in certain birds though there appear to be no T-tubules. In similar vein is the observation that junctional processes have sometimes been reported on the SR membrane facing away from the T-tubule (Sommer & Johnson,

1979; Sommer, 1982). In all these situations, the possibility that very fine T-tubules have been missed for technical reasons should not be ruled out.

The areas of surface sarcolemma which are coupled with cisterns of junctional SR include portions of the intercalated discs (Fig. 2.5). In the disc region the SR sacs are invariably related to the 'non-specialised' lengths of membrane, i.e. they are not related to nexuses, desmosomes, fasciae adherentes or interfibrillar regions. Most often the SR is found only on one side of the disc though, not infrequently, sacs may be seen on both sides.

The major protein component of SR membrane is the calcium pump (Blayney, 1983) but the actual mechanisms by which calcium makes its passage into and out of the SR lumen are still debatable; cytochemical studies by Malouf & Meissner (1984) confirm that $(Ca^{2+}Mg^{2+})$ ATPase is localised on the membrane of junctional SR. The intraluminal granules present as an electron-dense line which bisects the lumen of the junctional SR and Walker, Schrodt & Edge (1971) reported that these intraluminal densities have connections with the SR envelope which alternate with the junctional processes on the cytoplasmic side of the membrane. As regards the chemical nature of the granules, the evidence suggests that they are negatively charged proteins possibly representative of high-affinity calcium-

Fig. 4.5. Left ventricular myocardium of young adult rat labelled with horseradish peroxidase. Semi-thin section (0.5–1 μm) to demonstrate primary (T_1) and secondary (T_2) transverse tubules as well as longitudinal elements (T_L) of the T-system. The branch points are readily seen in this preparation. Picture by courtesy of Mr J.N. Skepper.

Fig. 4.6. Thin section of right atrial myocardium of young adult rat showing cisterns of junctional sarcoplasmic reticulum (SR) coupled with the surface plasma membrane. Note the luminal granules in the SR and the dense spicules attached to the SR membrane facing the sarcolemma.

Fig. 4.7. Thin section of the sinu-atrial node region of a young adult rat. Nodal cells (NC) are characterised by poor myofibrillae, absence of atrial granules and a poorly developed T-system. In transitional cells (TC), myofibrillae are better developed but granules and T-tubules are poorly represented.

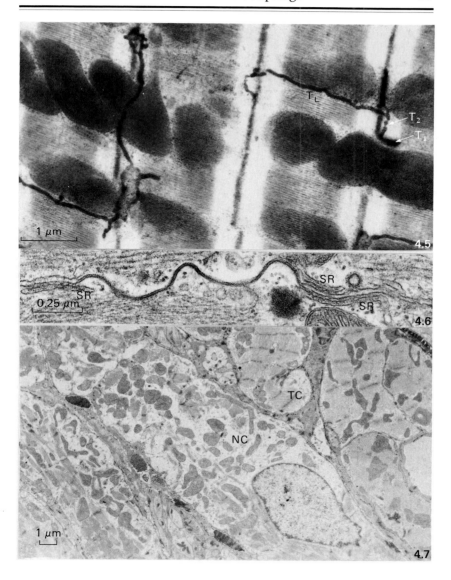

binding proteins including calsequestrin. Electron-probe microanalysis confirms that Ca^{2+} is normally localised in SR cisterns which become depleted by contracture induced by caffeine (Wendt-Galitelli, Stöhr, Wolburg & Schlote, 1980). The junctional membrane processes are projections measuring about 25–30 nm across, distributed in regular orthogonal array about $1000\,\mu m^{-2}$. There have been suggestions that these processes constitute a nexus-like low-resistance gap between SR and T-tubule (or sarcolemma) but most of the freeze-fracture and other ultrastructural analyses do not bear out this idea, for there appears to be no correspondence between (i) particles on the SR membrane, (ii) particles on the T-tubule membrane and (iii) junctional processes (Franzini-Armstrong, 1974; Smith, Baerwald & Hart, 1975) though Rayns, Devine & Sutherland (1975) have claimed that there is reasonably good correspondence between the distribution of particles on SR and T-tubule membranes. Forbes & Sperelakis (1977) favoured the view that junctional processes are conical elevations of the SR membrane but the fact that tilted views never reveal the appearance of unit membrane reduces the strength of such an interpretation.

Atrial myocardium

In typical atrial cells the presence of specific granules (see Chapter 6) may obscure the identification of peroxidase-filled tubules especially where these tubules are transected. However, peroxidase staining is usually darker than granule material and, moreover, in preparations where lengths of tubules appear, it is possible to gain a comprehensive picture of the T-system.

The T-system in atrial cells is less extensive than in general ventricular myocardium. It comprises primary T-tubules and longitudinal tubules but very few secondary or tertiary T-tubules can be identified. The primary tubules measure about 105 nm in diameter, which is narrower than in ventricular cells. They are invaginated from the sarcolemma and lie at I-band level close to the Z-line. There are numerous couplings with the SR at this level. Longitudinal tubules in atrial cells are similar in size and distribution to those in the ventricle in that they measure about 67 nm in diameter and run along the length of a single sarcomere from one set of primary invaginations towards the next; several couplings with the SR can be identified along the way. Couplings between SR sacs and sarcolemma are also present at the surface of the atrial cell and at intercalated discs. The features of all couplings are very similar to those seen in the ventricle; intraluminal granules are present in the SR and the cytoplasmic gap containing junctional processes, between the constituent membranes, is about 10–12 nm.

Sinu-atrial node

Sinu-atrial (SA) nodal cells are distinguishable from general atrial myocardium by their small size, their poorly developed and irregularly arranged content of myofibrillae and by the absence of specific atrial granules in their cytoplasm (Fig. 4.7). Moreover, compared to general myocardial cells, the T-system is poorly defined even in peroxidase-treated material. There are short, narrow (about 60 nm in diameter) invaginations of the sarcolemma which probably correspond to primary T-tubules, but they are far less regular than in typical atrial or ventricular cells, and even those that are present do not usually penetrate sufficiently far to contact the myofibrillae. A similarly restricted system was reported by Challice (1965) in the rabbit SA node and by Colborn & Carsey (1972) in the squirrel monkey. The primary invaginations do not give off any branches and, moreover, couplings between them and the SR have not been identified. The SR itself is not a prominent feature, but some peripherally lying sacs coupled with the sarcolemma can be identified. Typical intercalated discs do not occur in the SA node; most of the cell-to-cell contact is made by unspecialised sarcolemma (there are occasional desmosomes and a few punctate nexuses) and SR couplings occur as frequently in relation to cell contacts as anywhere else on the surface.

There are several transitional cells within the SA node and immediately surrounding it which, though they resemble nodal cells in diminutiveness of size and in lack of atrial granule, possess better developed T-system, SR and myofibrillae. They contain primary T-tubules and longitudinal tubules with SR couplings similar to those found in the general atrial musculature.

Atrioventricular node

The ultrastructural features of typical cells in the atrioventricular (AV) node are in many ways similar to those of SA nodal cells in that they are small and spindle-shaped with sparsely distributed myofibrillae and no atrial granules. Moreover, they lack typical intercalated discs, the cell contacts being predominantly of unspecialised membrane with a few desmosomes and occasional punctate nexuses.

The T-system in these cells is limited to short, narrow invaginations; they enter into couplings with the SR, a feature which has not been observed in the SA node. There are no longitudinal or other branches of the primary tubules, and the SR itself is poorly differentiated apart from sub-sarcolemmal sacs which have typical couplings with the surface membrane at cell junctions and elsewhere. James & Sherf (1968) reported similar findings in the human AV node.

In the postero-inferior part of the interatrial septum, just behind the AV node, there are cells which are intermediate in appearance between typical atrial myocardial cells and typical nodal cells. Like nodal cells they are small, spindle-shaped and lack specific atrial granules but they contain a better developed T-system and SR. Such cells are generally termed atrio-nodal cells or prenodal cells and their T-system comprises primary T-tubules and longitudinal branches similar to the arrangement found in atrial myocardium, though the longitudinal elements are narrower (44 nm). Couplings between the SR and T-system are frequently encountered. In many respects therefore atrio-nodal cells resemble transitional sinu-atrial cells.

Atrioventricular bundle and bundle branches

There is no sharp demarcation between the AV node and the bundle. Nevertheless, as one passes from node to bundle and then to bundle branches, the cells increase in diameter, the myofibrillae become more prominent and more regularly arranged, while intercalated discs, which include nexuses and interfibrillary regions as well as desmosomes and unspecialised membrane, can be recognised with increasing frequency. Bundle cells have a moderately well developed T-system which comprises primary T-tubules measuring about 72 nm in diameter and longitudinal branches of approximately 46 nm in diameter; both these components, but particularly the primary invaginations, are associated with SR couplings. Couplings of SR with sarcolemma along the free surface of the cells and along unspecialised parts of intercalated discs are also frequently observed. No secondary or tertiary T-tubules have been observed in bundle cells. Hayashi (1971) could not find a T-tubule system in the conducting system in the dog, nor could Kim & Baba (1971) in the guinea-pig, Virágh & Porte (1973) in the monkey or Mochet, Moravec, Guillemot & Hatt (1975) in the rat. On the other hand, James, Sherf & Urthaler (1974) found a restricted system comprising only primary tubules in human bundle branches.

Terminal ramifications of bundle branches

It is not always possible to distinguish between terminal muscle fibres of the AV conducting system and general ventricular cells. However, as a rule, the former cells are considerably thicker and may have a diameter of almost 26 μm, compared with a mean diameter of 16 μm for ventricular myocardial cells. SR and myofibrillae are generally well developed so that these features may not be useful in the recognition of terminal ramifications. However, a consistent feature is the presence of longer nexuses in intercalated discs within these ramifications when compared with the surrounding myocardium.

The T-system is less well developed than in other parts of the ventricle wall. The primary invaginations (102 nm in diameter) are not quite as wide and there are few secondary T-tubules and, where these occur, they are very narrow (about 40 nm in diameter). On the other hand, longitudinal branches are frequent and they are fairly wide (62 nm). Tertiary T-tubules could not be identified. Couplings between T-tubules and SR are common, especially at primary tubules and, in addition, frequent couplings occur between peripherally lying sacs of SR and the sarcolemma, including the intercalated disc regions. Sommer & Johnson (1968a,b) could find no T-tubules in the Purkinje system of the mouse heart, nor could Hayashi (1971) in the dog, whereas Page (1967b) identified primary T-tubules in the cat.

Implications of the distribution of T-tubules and SR couplings

From the studies on peroxidase-infiltrated material, it does appear that the T-system is a general feature of all myocardial cells in the rat but its degree of differentiation varies in different parts of the heart. It is modestly, or even poorly, represented in the specialised impulse-generating and conducting tissue especially in the nodes while it is a prominent feature of working myocardium particularly in the ventricular wall.

The sequence of excitation–contraction coupling in skeletal muscle cells is believed to entail transmission of excitation from the surface membrane to the interior along the T-tubule membrane. The mechanism whereby the signal is conveyed along the T-tubule membrane is not entirely clear, early evidence favouring the view that it occurs by passive cable-like transmission rather than by propagation of the action potential. Later results from voltage clamp experiments indicated that in skeletal muscle regenerative propagation of action potential along T-tubule membranes does occur, and that it is probably essential for the initiation of contraction (see Bastian & Nakajima, 1974). Depolarisation affects the terminal cisterns of SR whence it is thought to release Ca^{2+} which diffuses to the nearby myofibrillae to activate the troponin sites on actin filaments thus initiating the contractile mechanism. Contraction is believed to be terminated by an active ATP-driven calcium sequestration into the longitudinal tubules of the SR from whence it is translocated back to the terminal cisterns. The SR at couplings has certainly been shown to contain Ca^{2+} ATPase activity as well as Ca^{2+} itself (see Forbes & Sperelakis, 1977), but the precise manner in which calcium release from the SR is effected is not clear. Two possible mechanisms have been suggested, namely: (1) depolarisation of the SR membrane – this is regarded as the most likely mechanism in skeletal muscle (Baylor & Oetliker, 1975; Bezanilla & Horowicz, 1975; Natori, 1975; Endo, 1977); and (2) the slow entry of Ca^{2+} into the cell from the extracellular space, which is known to occur during activation of the sarcolemma, is thought to trigger the release of larger quantities of Ca^{2+} from the SR (see Fabiato, 1977).

By means of voltage clamp experiments, it has been demonstrated that some calcium enters myocardial cells during depolarisation in the order of 1×10^{-6} mol/kg of cell per beat. Cardiac muscle is more sensitive to the effects of slow Ca^{2+} inflow than skeletal muscle and calcium-induced calcium release from the SR is thought to be more easily evoked. Lüllman, Peters & Preuner (1983), however, deny that there are sufficient stores of Ca^{2+} in the SR of cardiac muscle for the purpose and they favour the view that there is a high affinity binding site at the inner surface of the sarcolemma which releases Ca^{2+} upon depolarisation and binds Ca^{2+} upon repolarisation (see Langer, Frank & Philipson, 1982, and Noble, 1983, for reviews of possible interrelationships between membrane systems in the cardiac cell concerned with Ca^{2+} movement).

A feature of cardiac muscle not shared by skeletal muscle is the presence of numerous couplings between surface sarcolemma and peripherally lying SR sacs. Whether or not this feature is designed to boost the effects of slow calcium entry through the sarcolemma during depolarisation is arguable, but it is striking that such peripheral couplings are present in all types of myocardial cell, even in SA nodal cells which lack deeper coupling arrangements.

Huxley & Taylor (1958) showed in skeletal muscle that contraction and local activation of the SR via a single T-invagination was confined to the adjacent half sarcomeres, which suggested that calcium was released only from the adjacent coupled terminal cisternae. This interpretation received support from the autoradiographical studies of Winegrad (1970) which indicated that calcium is released physiologically mainly from the terminal cisterns, where the main part of calcium is stored in resting muscle. On the other hand, for cardiac muscle, Müller showed that localised surface stimulation does not elicit localised contraction but instead causes widespread contraction of practically all the sarcomeres in the field of observation. A possible explanation of Müller's findings is that the distribution of couplings in typical cardiac muscle is far more extensive than in skeletal muscle, for it includes some at every level of an extensive T-system as well as others in relation to the surface sarcolemma. Moreover, the SR is not separated into units corresponding to each sarcomere, but extends across Z-line levels by narrow but distinct cisterns.

Hamster myocardium

The ultrastructure of the myocardium, including the specialised nodal and conducting systems, was studied in adult golden hamsters *Mesocricetus auratus* of the WO strain.

Ventricular myocardium

The ventricular myocardial cells measure 12–18 µm in diameter and, in addition to a centrally located nucleus, each contains prominent myofibrillae, mitochondria, SR, Golgi apparatus and glycogen granules as well as several large lipid bodies. However, the most striking feature is the presence of exceptionally wide T-tubules (Figs. 4.8, 4.9). There are numerous primary T-tubule invaginations of the sarcolemma projecting towards the I-bands of the

Fig. 4.8. Electron micrograph of right ventricular myocardium of a golden hamster showing large T-tubules, with a prominent lining of basement membrane. L, lipid droplet.

Fig. 4.9. Left ventricular myocardium of a golden hamster showing a large longitudinal element (T_L) of the T-system which is coupled with an SR cistern. Note the caveolae (c) budding off the T-system.

Fig. 4.10. Freeze-fracture replica of right ventricular myocardium of a golden hamster, showing primary T-tubules and SR network. M, mitochondria.

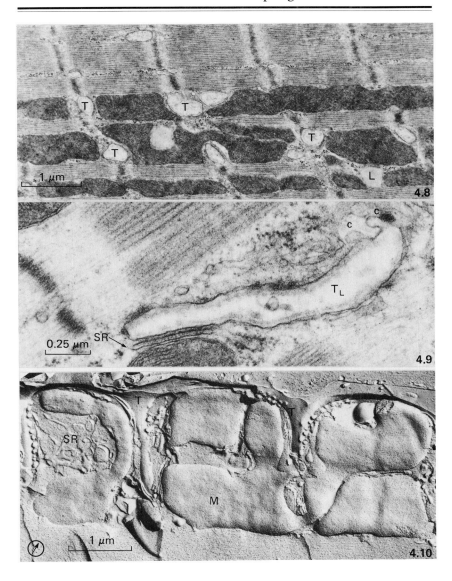

4.8

4.9

4.10

myofibrillae (Fig. 4.10). These primary tubules measure about 450–500 nm across and contain a clearly identifiable luminal coating of basement membrane. Narrower branches measuring 200–250 nm arise from the primary tubules, some ramifying in the transverse plane across the I-band region (secondary T-tubules) and others running longitudinally towards the primary tubules at the opposite end of the sarcomere (Figs. 4.9, 4.11). Cross-connections between the longitudinal elements at A-band level cannot be discerned, i.e. there is no evidence of tertiary tubules. All levels of the T-system, but particularly the primary invaginations, show couplings with the SR. The SR at such coupling sites has the typical structure of junctional cisterns containing fine luminal granules which are not present in the remaining free SR (Fig. 4.9). The cytoplasmic gap between the membranes of the T-tubule and SR is about 10 nm and there are electron-dense processes projecting from the SR membrane towards, but not quite contacting, the T-tubule. Couplings of similar nature are found between superficial cisterns of SR and the surface sarcolemma, including the sarcolemma of intercalated discs.

Atrial myocardium

Atrial myocytes are more slender (8–11 μm in diameter) than ventricular cells. The primary T-tubules measure about 250 nm in diameter and form couplings with SR near the I-band region of myofibrillae. No longitudinal branches can be observed and T–SR couplings appear to be restricted to the vicinity of I-bands. However, there are numerous couplings between the SR and surface sarcolemma, including portions of intercalated discs.

Fig. 4.11. Freeze-fracture replica of hamster right ventricular myocardium showing prominent longitudinal elements (T_L) of the T-system.

Fig. 4.12. Thin section of right ventricular myocardium of a fruit-eating bat showing large primary T-tubules (T) coupled with cisterns of sarcoplasmic reticulum (SR) and one of them gives off a prominent longitudinal branch (T_L) running alongside myofibrillae.

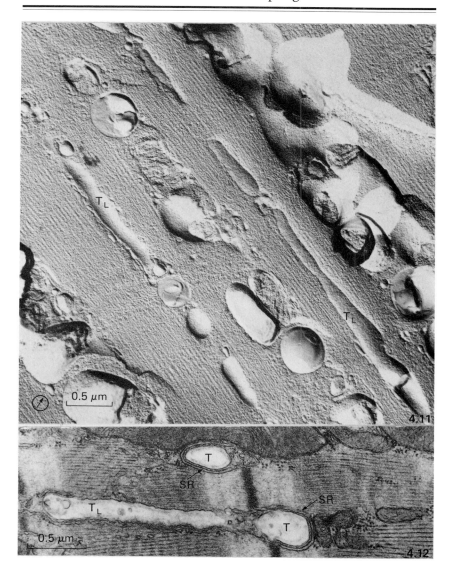

Nodal and conducting systems

The cells of the sinu-atrial and atrioventricular nodes are small (about 6–8 μm in diameter) and spindle-shaped. Myofibrillae are few and irregularly aligned and the cells lack the specific granules which are characteristic of working atrial myocardium. No T-tubules could be found in the nodal cells but surface couplings between SR and sarcolemma are present.

In the atrioventricular bundle and its distal ramifications, the myocytes are larger than in the nodes but nowhere are they larger than in general ventricular myocardial cells. Myofibrillae are more prominent and become more regularly aligned as one passes down the bundle and its branches and the T-system also becomes correspondingly enhanced.

The functional significance of wide T-tubules, especially the primary invaginations, in the working myocardium of the golden hamster is not clear. Other species with unusually large T-tubules include diving seals (Ayettey & Navaratnam, 1980) and bats (Fig. 4.12 and see Navaratnam *et al.*, 1986*a*) and it is of interest that all these species share the capacity for a substantial variation in heart rate. Hamsters have a normal heart rate of about 450/min which can fall to 4–15/min during hibernation (Spector, 1956) when the temperature may fall to 5°C without ventricular arrhythmia. A diving seal such as the grey seal (*Halichoerus grypus*) shows range in heart rate from 120/min to 4/min during diving (Harrison & Ridgway, 1976). Several species of bat show the capacity for dormancy while some do enter true hibernation; their range in physical activity from dormancy or hibernation to active flight calls for extensive variations in heart rate. It is possible, of course, that the large size of T-tubules in these species represents a coincidence of little functional significance but it is worth considering whether the presence of wide T-tubules has a protective role during extreme bradycardia. It could be a mechanism to ensure that excitation–contraction remains effective at low heart rates or it could represent a simple increase in surface area for transport across the cell membrane.

———

In the typical mammalian myocardium, primary T-tubules are invaginations of the sarcolemma at or near Z-line level. They give off transverse branches or secondary T-tubules, which form a network in relation to the I-bands on either side of the Z-line, as well as longitudinal branches which run alongside the myofibrillae. The longitudinal tubules may be linked by narrow cross-channels (tertiary T-tubules) at A-band level. All levels of the T-system may show coupling arrangements with cisterns of SR which are believed to be related to the excitation–contraction sequence, and similar couplings are also found in relation to the surface sarcolemma. At such couplings the SR is modified (junctional SR) in that it contains intraluminal granules, which probably contain calcium-binding proteins including calsequestrin, and membrane projections which protrude into the cytoplasm towards the T-tubule or sarcolemma.

The T-system is widest and most extensive in ventricular myocytes but it is also fairly well expressed in the general atrial myocardium. It is poorly represented in the sinu-atrial and atrioventricular nodes where SR couplings are mainly restricted to the sarcolemma. The T-system varies in the conducting system, being poor at the atrial end of the bundle but extensive in the ventricular ramifications of the bundle branches.

In most terrestrial species, such as the rat, primary T-tubules measure about 100–150 nm in diameter. In contrast, in bats, diving seals and hamsters, the T-system is exceptionally wide and the primary tubules range from 350 to 500 nm in diameter; these species are seemingly unrelated but they all possess the capacity for wide variation in heart rate during the physiological states associated with flying, diving or hibernation.

5

Endogenous substrates – lipid droplets and glycogen particles. Effects of ischaemic arrest on myocardial ultrastructure

In several varieties of cell, the intermediary metabolic pathways generate storage products that are readily visible under the electron microscope. The most visually obvious examples of such products in cardiac myocytes, as well as the most important, are triglyceride fat droplets (the storage form of fatty acids) and glycogen which is the major storage form of carbohydrate. That these inclusions contribute towards energy production is shown by the observation that both lipid droplets and glycogen particles are depleted in heart muscle preparations made to contract without exogenous substrate and, indeed, glycogen is depleted even if exogenous substrates are provided.

Lipid droplets

In myocardial tissue, fatty acids are present in the unesterified (NEFA) and esterified (EFA) forms. NEFA accounts for less than 0.1% of total fatty acids in normoxic dog myocardium (van der Vusse & Reneman, 1983) but values reported in the literature show substantial variations even in the same species possibly because of varying anaesthetic procedures, feeding schedules and differences in experimental conditions; they are predominantly bound to proteins or other components of the cytosol compartment of sarcoplasm. On the other hand, esterified fatty acids are present as phosphoglycerides (about 85%), triacylglycerols (14%), di- and mono-esterified glycerols and cholesteryl esters (0.5%).

The main function of phosphoglycerides is as essential components of biological membranes and, although they are subject to a continuous turnover process, there is good evidence that they do not constitute a store of fatty acids available for mitochondrial energy production. The function of the relatively small amount of cholesteryl esters in myocardial cells is yet to be clarified but a possible role as endogenous substrate is not considered likely.

Triacylglycerol, which has a high calorie value of $9 \, kcal \, g^{-1}$, is the most likely candidate for the endogenous lipid store. Insoluble triglycerides coalesce in the cytosol as anhydrous lipid droplets and they are also thought to be stored in lysosomes (Hülsmann & Stam, 1979). Electron micrographs of cardiac myocytes reveal typical round droplets without a limiting membrane (Figs. 5.1, 5.2, 5.3, 5.4). They are roughly the same size in all species and they comprise homogenous electron-lucent material which may be leached out in material where acetone has been used in the dehydrating process. They are closely apposed to mitochondria which they frequently indent (Figs. 5.2, 5.4) and are often found where mitochondria lie close to junctional SR and T-tubules. The possibility that triacylglycerol is also stored in smaller aggregates, not directly discernible in electron micrographs, should also be considered (Masters & Glaviano, 1972). Natural abundance ^{13}C NMR spectra of perfused guinea-pig hearts reveal sharp peaks, particularly in the $-C=C-$ and $-CH_2-$ backbone regions, which must originate from mobile components including lipids contained in the droplets (P.F. Morris, personal communication).

In contrast with the varied values reported in the literature for NEFA content of myocardial cells, there appears to be good agreement for triacylglycerol content. Assuming a mean triacylglycerol content of $2 \, \mu mol \, g^{-1}$ the normal energy requirements can be met for about 38 min when the heart depends solely on endogenous fat; in comparison, the NEFA content of heart muscle represents less than ten seconds of myocardial performance although the normal major metabolic substrates for cardiac muscle are glucose, lactate and circulating NEFA.

Though lipid droplets in different species are of similar size, their numerical density varies from species to species. Moreover, there is variation between the musculature of different chambers in the same species. For instance, Bruce & Myers (1973) reported that the lipid content of right ventricular muscle in the dog exceeds that of the left ventricle. On the other hand, morphometric observations on the rat, hamster and mouse suggest that the right ventricular myocardium is comparable to that of the left ventricle in regard to droplet content but that the content in either ventricle wall exceeds that in atrial muscle by a factor of five or ten.

Comparative studies of corresponding chambers in different species show a striking difference between the myocardium of typical terrestrial mammals such as the rat or the mouse and that of flying species like the bat *Eidolon helvum* and of hibernating species like the golden hamster (Navaratnam et al., 1986a). The proportional volume of right ventricular myocytes (Table 5.1) occupied by droplets in the bat (0.0365 ± 0.007) is over ten times that in the rat (0.0029 ± 0.001). The wide range of physiological activity exhibited by bats, from high exercise tolerance to dormancy or even hibernation in some varieties, makes it likely that there are adaptive features in the cardio-pulmonary and other systems. Ultrastructural observations confirm that there are adaptations in the fine structure of cardiac myocytes comprising larger fractional volumes not only of lipid droplets but also of mitochondria and T-tubules. It is possible that the prominence of lipid droplets is associated with the enhanced dependence on endogenous fatty acid metabolism for energy requirements during flight as similarly increased numbers of lipid droplets are present in the cardiac myocytes of birds. Such a view is also supported by the intimate relationship between lipid, T-tubules and SR as both the latter organelles have been implicated in the formation and transport of triacylglycerides (Stein & Stein, 1971).

Nevertheless, there are non-flying species in which cardiac myocytes possess an enhanced content of lipid in the form of droplets. They include the golden hamster (Ayettey & Navaratnam, 1981) where both ventricular and atrial myocytes contain substantially more droplet lipid than their counterparts in the rat (Table 5.1 and Figs. 5.1, 5.2). This suggests that there could be explanations other

Fig. 5.1. Thin section of left ventricular myocardium of adult golden hamster showing numerous lipid droplets (L).

Fig. 5.2. Detailed view of lipid droplets (L) in left ventricular myocyte of golden hamster showing their close apposition to mitochondria and to the sarcoplasmic reticulum (SR).

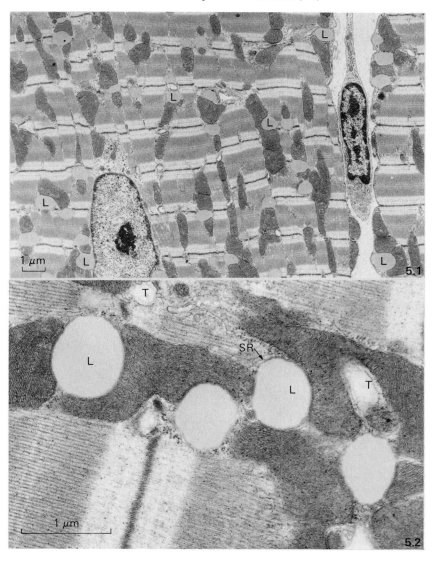

than exercise tolerance for increased lipid storage products. Many bats exhibit torpor and some varieties, such as the big brown bat, are true hibernators like the hamster. During hibernation, animals are known to depend heavily on lipid metabolism (Fonda, Herbener & Cuddihee, 1983) and it is possible that this capacity as well as high exercise tolerance contribute to the presence of lipid droplets in increased numbers (Figs. 5.3, 5.4).

Reduction in the oxygen supply to the heart results in impaired myocardial performance and in changes of carbohydrate and lipid metabolism. It has been claimed that among the effects of oxygen restriction are depletion of glycogen and accumulation of tri-acylglycerol in myocardial cells (Kloner, Fishbein, Hare & Maroko,

Fig. 5.3. Electron micrograph of right ventricular myocyte in a fruit-eating bat showing a large lipid droplet (L) closely apposed to a mitochondrion (M), to a cistern of sarcoplasmic reticulum (SR) and to a secondary T-tubule (T_2). Note also the large primary T-tubule (T_1) coupled with another SR cistern.

Fig. 5.4. Right ventricular myocyte of fruit-eating bat showing two lipid droplets (L), indenting mitochondria (M). One droplet is closely apposed to a cistern of SR.

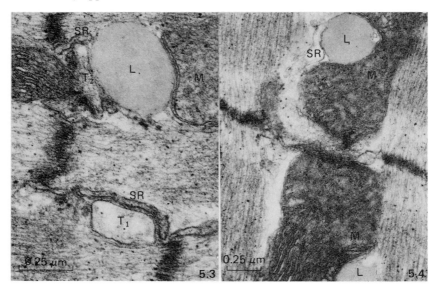

Table 5.1 *Proportions of myocyte volume (mean values ± s.e.)
occupied by different organelles and myoplasm in the right
ventricular myocardium of rat, hamster and bat*

	T-tubules	Mitochondria	Lipid droplets	Myofibrillae	Myoplasm
Rat	0.0130 ± 0.002 (23)	0.282 ± 0.015 (505)	0.0029 ± 0.001 (5)	0.655 ± 0.023 (1201)	0.05 (90)
Hamster	0.0369 ± 0.005 (88)	0.322 ± 0.016 (762)	0.0310 ± 0.006 (70)	0.577 ± 0.019 (1349)	0.03 (79)
Bat	0.0405 ± 0.003 (93)	0.411 ± 0.011 (929)	0.0365 ± 0.007 (81)	0.473 ± 0.010 (1078)	0.04 (96)

Figures in parentheses indicate the number of hits scored on the relevant organelles in 9
micrographs of material taken from 3 individual animals from each species. Cumulative
mean error was not more than ± 10% for any feature and in most instances was less
than ± 3% suggesting that the differences revealed by this preliminary survey are
significant.

1979). Opie *et al.* (1973) have reported that circulating NEFA
competes unfavourably with glucose for residual oxygen in
ischaemic hearts as a result of which there is more NEFA for
esterification. Be that as it may, histochemical studies have shown
that there is a virtually unchanged net content of triacylglycerol
during the first two hours of ischaemia although key precursor
substances such as α-glycerol phosphate may be increased several-
fold over the same period.

Glycogen particles

Large highly-branched molecules of glycogen appear as very dark
cytoplasmic granules in electron micrographs (Figs. 5.5, 5.6).
Cardiac muscle, like skeletal muscle contains relatively large
quantities of such particles only exceeded by liver cells, and glycogen content is said to be capable of providing about 1% of the
energy required by cardiac myocytes although there is some species
variation. Most of it is found in the form of β-granules which are
smooth and ovoid measuring about 30 nm in diameter and some of
these granules show a substructure of rod-like elements, sometimes
termed γ-particles. They are usually dispersed as separate granules

(Figs. 5.5, 5.6) but a small proportion are grouped to form conglomerates or α-particles, 80–120 nm in diameter (Fig. 5.7). Such conglomerates are relatively rare in muscle but they form the majority of glycogen particles in liver cells. In cardiac myocytes, glycogen is mainly concentrated along the mitochondrial columns between myofibrillae but it is also present in the perinuclear sarcoplasm and near SR including the sub-sarcolemmal cisterns. When found near myofibrillae the particles tend to lie apposed to I-bands.

Glycogen stains heavily with lead but it can be demonstrated more specifically by cytochemical techniques such as the thiosemicarbazide-silver proteinate or the periodic acid-bismuth methods (see Lewis & Knight, 1977). Ultrastructural studies give variable results because the preservation depends on the fixation and subsequent treatment of tissue. Thus statements about the metabolic status of cardiac muscle based on ultrastructural estimates of

Fig. 5.5. Electron micrograph of ventricular myocardium of 5-month human foetus (130 mm C.R.) showing a vast number of glycogen granules of the β type in the myocyte cytoplasm.

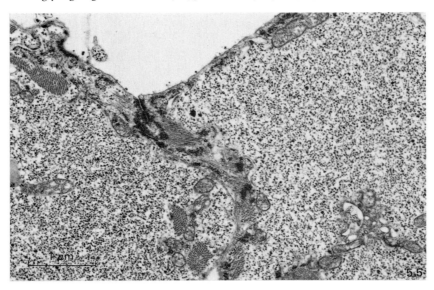

Fig. 5.6. Enlargement of Fig. 5.5 showing β-particles of glycogen in human foetal ventricular myocyte.

Fig. 5.7. Electron micrograph of atrioventricular bundle myocyte from an adult golden hamster, to show glycogen (Gly) in β-particle and α-particle form.

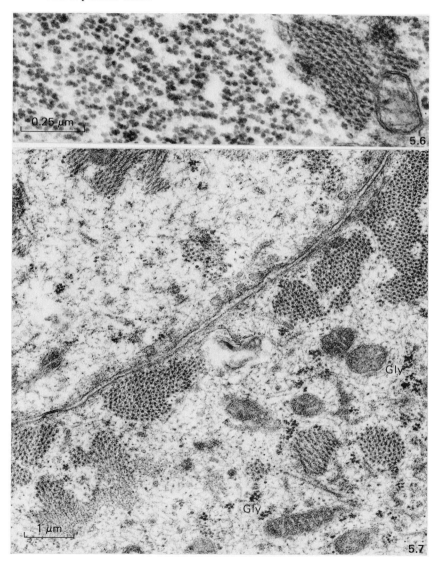

glycogen particles should be treated with caution (see below). Glycogen is well preserved by hypertonic fixatives such as Karnovsky's mixture of aldehydes whereas bulk staining with uranyl acetate provides unreliable results (Virágh & Challice, 1973).

Detailed analysis of glycogen β-granules indicates that the core contains the glycogen molecule arranged in the form of branched chains of glucose residues coupled by extensive linkages. This is enclosed in a monolayer of enzyme molecules bound to the surface and they include the synthetic enzyme glycogen synthase and the degradative enzyme glycogen phosphatase.

In specialised nodal cells and in the atrioventricular conducting system, there is a greater proportion of sarcoplasm unoccupied by larger organelles such as myofibrillae, mitochondria and T-tubules and as a result glycogen particles are more easily recognised in these clear areas (Fig. 5.7). This probably accounts for the many descriptions in the classical light-microscopic literature (Aschoff, 1908; Ungar, 1924; Schiebler, 1955) of enhanced glycogen content in such specialised cells. On the other hand, ultrastructural studies show that the glycogen content in working myocardial cells is highly variable and that the characteristically slender cells in the nodes and in the atrioventricular bundle contain no more glycogen than the surrounding myocardium though it is more easily visualised (Virágh & Challice, 1973). Some ultrastructural descriptions claim that a proportion of nodal cells are larger and clearer than others and that they contain more glycogen (see Sommer & Johnson, 1979). The claim that nodal and bundle cells contain enhanced levels of glycogen is still unproven but, in those species containing typically enlarged Purkinje cells as in ungulate hearts (see Nandy & Bourne, 1963; Chiodi & Bartolami, 1967), the evidence for enhanced glycogen content in these cells is more convincing (see Virágh & Challice, 1973).

In view of the necessity to protect heart muscle during surgical procedures, it is of importance to consider the effects of acute reduction of myocardial blood flow on glycogen content among other features. Reduction of oxygen supply to the heart *in vivo* and *in vitro* is said to result in depletion of glycogen and the majority of ultrastructural observations support this view (see below).

Experimental studies using ^{13}C NMR spectroscopy have been applied to isolated ischaemic hearts whereby it has been possible to evaluate glycogen and lactate levels in the heart and to correlate these with ^{31}P NMR studies which monitor ATP, inorganic phosphate and pH levels. The findings indicate that glycogen levels fall and that lactate levels rise during ischaemia concurrent with degradation of CP, slower phosphorylation of ATP, lowering of pH and accumulation of inorganic phosphate.

Repair of intracardiac defects and the insertion of coronary bypass grafts require a static and practically bloodless operating field. To this purpose, cross-clamping of the ascending aorta is usually applied resulting in an ischaemically arrested heart while the systemic blood supply is maintained by extracorporeal circulation. Van der Vusse & Reneman (1983) report that in the human heart glycogen content is reduced during ischaemia and they advocate the monitoring of glycogen content to assess the value of cardioprotective regimes. Some authorities emphasise the importance of pre-operative myocardial glycogen levels in cardiac preservation (Lolley *et al.*, 1979). Protection by raising pre-operative myocardial glycogen is thought to be more important when cardiac arrest is effected at relatively high body temperatures (25°–34°C) when considerable energy requirements still persist. On the other hand, it is not certain that it has any significant value when complete anoxic arrest is effected in combination with the use of cold, high-potassium cardioplegic solutions.

EFFECTS OF ISCHAEMIC ARREST ON MYOCARDIAL ULTRASTRUCTURE

The capacity of the heart to survive ischaemic arrest and to resume function has been crucial in the development of cardiac transplantation and also of cardiac surgery when a still and bloodless field is required. The following section is devoted to ultrastructural changes which have been observed during and after ischaemic arrest as well as to protective procedures aimed at circumventing such myocardial damage. For transplant purposes it is contemporary practice to arrest the donor heart by coronary infusion of a cold cardioplegic solution following cross-clamping of the aorta and, after removal, it is placed in a cold protective medium for transfer; some authorities suggest that perfusion or intermittent flushing of the coronary bed with either whole blood or a protective electrolyte solution may be beneficial during the ischaemic period (see Losman, 1980, for a description of transplantation procedure and for a résumé of the historical background) though the circumstances of human heart transplantation seldom favour such a procedure. After transplantation, reperfusion occurs as the heart resumes function. In cardiac surgery too, ischaemic arrest is usually effected by coronary infusion of a cold cardioplegic solution following cross-clamping of the aorta. The patient is put on cardio-pulmonary bypass, principally to protect the brain, while the heart is rendered bloodless and further protection of the myocardium may be afforded by systemic and topical hypothermia and by coronary perfusion with blood or asanguineous solution (see Hearse, Braimbridge & Jynge, 1981).

The effects of ischaemic arrest on the human myocardium are not easy to evaluate accurately although several investigators have conducted invaluable studies by taking biopsies during the arrested phase and after reperfusion (Fischer & Barner, 1978; Nonoyama *et al.*, 1978; Shiraishi *et al.*, 1980; Schaper, Stämmler & Scheld, 1981; Lindal, Myklebust, Sørlie & Jørgensen, 1983; Takimoto *et al.*, 1983; Görlach *et al.*, 1986). However, such biopsy material can be processed by immersion fixation only and, despite the great care taken during fixation, the variability of preservation within the same sample and between samples is such that it interferes with the proper interpretation of ultrastructure. On the other hand, animal experiments allow perfusion fixation which yields uniform and more reliable preservation (see Jynge *et al.*, 1978) though the increased attention required renders such investigations relatively cumbersome. Sanan, van der Merwe & Lochner (1985) conducted a comparison of glutaraldehyde immersion and perfusion fixation of rat heart muscle and found that immersion fixation tends to produce myofibrillar contracture, interfibrillar oedema and mitochondrial changes thus confusing the possible true sequellae of ischaemia; perfusion fixation, on the other hand, causes little or no damage. Some very interesting experiments, such as those by Menz *et al.* (1984) on orthotopically transplanted dog hearts and by Balderman, Binette, Chan & Gage (1983) on the protective effects of myocardial cooling could have been even more valuable had perfusion fixation been used for ultrastructural assessment.

Effects of normothermic ischaemic arrest

It is desirable to separate the consequences of ischaemia from any protective effects of cardioplegic solutions or hypothermia. To this end, the effects of global ischaemia have been studied in many experiments after cross-clamping of the aorta. Langendorff-type perfusion preparations, using an isolated heart and avoiding cardio-pulmonary bypass, have been used for similar purposes; the heart is capable of continuous pulsation in such preparations but can be arrested by clamping the aortic cannula. The consequences of partial ischaemia have also been investigated by restricting individual coronary arteries. The majority of reports demonstrate that, unless the heart is afforded protection, alterations in myocyte ultrastructure commence within a few minutes of ischaemia. Early subcellular changes in cardiac myocytes may involve mitochondria, glycogen granules, the sarcolemma, the nucleus, and lipid droplets as well as intracellular and extracellular oedema. Subsequently, there may be swelling and vacuolation of SR and T-tubules, disruption of sarcolemma and alterations in myofibrillar pattern and some of these later manifestations are thought to indicate irreversible change. However, many of the early subcellular changes can be reversed if reperfusion is effected within a period of about one half to one hour but reperfusion itself may exacerbate some changes and may induce new damage (see p. 117). Structural changes caused by ischaemia are most profound in the sub-endocardial zone of myocardium (Ashraf, White & Bloor, 1978;

Sunamori *et al.*, 1978; Shiraishi *et al.*, 1980; Uchida *et al.*, 1980; Edonte *et al.*, 1983) and they are not as easily reversed here as in other layers because this zone is less amenable to reflow (Gavin, Thomson, Humphrey & Herdson, 1983).

Mitochondria

Mitochondrial ultrastructure is widely accepted to be the most sensitive indicator of early ischaemic damage (Lochner *et al.*, 1986). The commonest manifestations are swelling and deformation of the organelle with disruption of cristae and the appearance of electron-dense deposits in the matrix (Harden *et al.*, 1978; Jynge *et al.*, 1978; Nayler, Gran & Yepez, 1978; Sunamori *et al.*, 1978; Kloner, Fishbein, Hare & Maroko, 1979; Uchida *et al.*, 1980; Slade & Nayler, 1981; De Boer *et al.*, 1983; Torok, Trombitás & Röth, 1983; Sashida & Abiko, 1986) and some of these changes, including mitochondrial swelling, can be reversed if reperfusion is effected within about one hour of ischaemic arrest (Schaper, Pinkowski & Froede, 1982). Despite these reports of mitochondrial swelling, Goldstein & Murphy (1983) found no increase in the mitochondrial volume fraction and, in fact, McCallister, Daiello & Tyers (1978) observed a decline in the fraction indicating a reduction in mitochondrial number. Several authors have shown that there is depressed mitochondrial function during ischaemic arrest including diminution of oxidative enzyme activity and of oxygen uptake (Harden *et al.*, 1978; Kloner *et al.*, 1979; Edonte *et al.*, 1983).

Glycogen, lipid and high energy phosphates

Although Flameng *et al.* (1981) did report an increase in glycogen content, most electron-microscopic observations point to an early reduction of glycogen granules during myocardial ischaemia (Harden *et al.*, 1978; McCallister, Daiello & Tyers, 1978; Kloner *et al.*, 1979; Kloner *et al.*, 1981; De Boer *et al.*, 1983; Goldstein & Murphy, 1983; Herscher *et al.*, 1984; Sashida & Abiko, 1986) but cytosolic swelling probably exaggerates the apparent extent of depletion (Prinzen, 1982). There are also several reports of depletion of the high energy phosphate compounds ATP and CP (Kloner *et al.*, 1981; Edonte *et al.*, 1983; Balderman, Binette, Chan & Gage, 1983; Ruigrok *et al.*, 1985) and the potential survival of the myocardium probably depends on the extent to which these compounds are retained (see Kirklin & Barratt-Boyes, 1986).

Many reports indicate that lipid droplets increase in number during ischaemic arrest (Kloner *et al.*, 1979; Slade & Nayler, 1981; Goldstein & Murphy, 1983) but there is little agreement on the time required for this manifestation. In contrast, Opie *et al.* (1973), on the basis of histochemical studies, have claimed that there is no increase in the net content of triacylglycerols.

Sarcolemma

Some authors regard the sarcolemma to be as sensitive to ischaemic arrest as mitochondria, but the changes may not be as easy to detect at early stages. Frank, Rich, Bedler & Kreman (1982) have described early separation of the glycocalyx and, in freeze-fracture preparations, a re-orientation of intramembranous particles, while Torok, Trombitás & Röth (1983) described a reduction in membrane thickness. Lochner *et al.* (1986) observed a reduction in cholesterol content and several authors have reported abnormal levels of creatine kinase leakage (Jynge *et al.*, 1978; Morgan, Bittner & Cohen, 1978; Ruigrot *et al.*, 1985). Later alterations, some of which probably indicate irreversible damage, include disruption of sarcolemmal continuity (Harden *et al.*, 1978; Nayler, Gran & Yepez, 1978) allowing abnormal permeability to extrinsic markers such as lanthanum (Ashraf, White & Bloor, 1978).

There is hardly any information about the state of nexuses or of cell-to-cell conduction during ischaemic arrest but, if changes do occur, satisfactory restoration of function by reperfusion indicates that they are reversible. Nevertheless, this seems to be a field worthy of more detailed exploration.

Other changes

Not all accounts refer to nuclear changes in ischaemic arrest but Uchida *et al.* (1980), Slade & Nayler (1981), De Boer *et al.* (1983) and Sashida & Abiko (1986) have claimed that margination and clumping of nuclear chromatin are frequent manifestations.

Cytosolic swelling has been observed by Kloner *et al.* (1979), Uchida *et al.* (1980) and Slade & Nayler (1981) and extracellular oedema has been described by Sunamori *et al.* (1978) and Uchida *et al.* (1980). Other authors, however, claim that oedema occurs only after reperfusion (Lindal, Mykleburst, Sørlie & Jørgensen, 1983; Prickaerts *et al.*, 1984); indeed, Schaper, Stämmler & Scheld (1981) contend that reperfusion is responsible not only for intracellular and extracellular oedema but also for mitochondrial swelling.

The most frequent alterations in myofibrillar pattern described during cardiac arrest comprise widening of the I-bands (Kloner *et al.*, 1981; De Boer *et al.*, 1983) but there are occasional descriptions of misalignment (Harden *et al.*, 1978) and gross disruption (Nayler, Gran & Yepez, 1978). More severe changes in myofibrillar organisation that may occur after reperfusion include changes in contractile bands, blurred Z-lines, rupture and lysis (Ashraf, White & Bloor, 1978; Torok, Trombitás & Röth, 1983; Humphrey, Thomson & Gavin, 1986; Humphrey & Vanderwee, 1986), and are frequently associated with disruption of intercalated discs.

Swelling or vacuolisation of SR and T-tubules have been described in the literature as fairly late sequellae of ischaemic arrest (McCallister, Daiello & Tyers, 1978; Kloner *et al.*, 1979; Slade & Nayler, 1981) and are held to be resistant to the restorative effects of reperfusion.

Protection by intermittent release of ischaemia

It has been claimed that intermittent ischaemia is a satisfactory and safe procedure which avoids myocardial damage. However Görlach *et al.* (1986), who studied the ultrastructure of the human myocardium after intermittent cross-clamping of the aorta during coronary surgery, found that severe and possibly irreversible damage had occurred although each ischaemic episode lasted only 6–20 min (mean: 10 min) and the total cross-clamping period was 75 ± 21 min. The principal feature of damage comprised intracellular oedema in myocytes and in capillary endothelium.

Protection by cooling

There is general agreement that lowering of myocardial temperature protects myocyte ultrastructure during ischaemic episodes mainly by reducing metabolic requirements and also probably by increasing the use of lactates, pyruvates and NEFA as energy fuels. The chief danger of hypothermia below 15°C is the high incidence of ventricular fibrillation but this problem can be mitigated by cardio-pulmonary bypass and by suitable cardioplegia which can provide a flaccid and inert heart. Myocardial cooling can be effected by a variable combination of systemic hypothermia and topical cooling by immersion or cold coronary perfusion.

Nonoyama et al. (1978) studied human clinical material as well as experimental dogs and concluded that, when the temperature is maintained below 15°C, structural integrity is well preserved during ischaemic arrest and there is only slight mitochondrial swelling and little glycogen loss. Shiraishi et al. (1980) found that topical cooling of the heart to 15°C with ice slush protects the myocardium from any structural damage for one hour after aortic cross-clamping and potassium cardioplegia. Even after 2.5 hours, the ultrastructural changes remain mild to moderate. Balderman et al. (1983) studied the effects of lowering myocardial temperature to various levels during global ischaemia and observed that satisfactory preservation of mitochondrial ultrastructure and retention of high energy phosphates are achieved below 18°C.

The findings summarised above do not reflect the protective effects of cooling alone because, in the relevant experiments, cardioplegia and coronary perfusion with blood or electrolyte solutions were employed to a variable degree. In a brief communication, Uchida et al. (1980) reported that cooling alone (whether effected topically or by a combination of topical and systemic hypothermia) is limited in its protective effect unless supplemented by intermittent or steady coronary perfusion.

Cardioplegia

The concept of cardioplegia or elective cardiac arrest for surgery was articulated about 1955 (see Hearse, Braimbridge & Jynge, 1981, for historical review) but, after a period of trial, it receded in popularity in the late 1960s and early 1970s. However, over the past ten years, cardioplegia with a cold hyperkalaemic solution has become standard procedure in most units; the raised potassium level causes arrest of the heart in diastole thus providing a temporarily flaccid and paralysed heart. Most authorities favour electrolyte cardioplegic solutions which offer the advantages of simplicity and lack of viscosity at low temperature but others (see Chen & Liu, 1984, for references) prefer blood as the cardioplegic vehicle because it provides oxygen and glucose and possesses a buffering capacity. Chen & Liu (1984) claimed that blood-potassium cardioplegia is more effective than a hyperkalaemic electrolyte solution in preserving the ultrastructure of human atrial myocardium.

Jynge *et al.* (1978) compared the effects of three electrolyte cardioplegic solutions, namely St Thomas (based on Ringer's solution, with normal extracellular concentration of sodium and calcium, to which potassium chloride and magnesium chloride were added), Bretschneider (high in potassium but moderate in sodium concentration, resembling the intracellular environment, and lacking calcium) and Kirsch (high in magnesium but lacking calcium, sodium and potassium) on rat hearts. From their findings, Jynge *et al.* concluded that the St Thomas solution affords the best protective effect especially in regard to potential reperfusion damage (see p. 117). At least part of this protective effect can be attributed to retention of some calcium in the St Thomas solution despite the known tendency for calcium to promote cardiac systole. The other two solutions are devoid of calcium, a state which renders the myocardium prone to damage when calcium is restored to the circulation; this phenomenon has been termed the calcium paradox. Similarly, Frank *et al.* (1982) found that the ultrastructure of cardiomyocyte sarcolemma can be protected by the addition of Ca^{2+} to the perfusate and possibly trace quantities are sufficient for this purpose (Øskendal, Jynge, Greve & Saetersdal, 1984). Moreover, Morgan, Bittner & Cohen (1978) claimed that Ca^{2+} protects against myocardial damage regardless of reperfusion. Sashida & Abiko (1986) found that diltiazem (a calcium channel blocker) also inhibits ultrastructural damage regardless of reperfusion. In contrast with the findings mentioned above, Görlach *et al.* (1986) observed no significant difference between the protective effects of the Bretschneider and St Thomas solutions. In recent years, the effects of using a cardioplegic solution, which combines the advantages of intracellular sodium levels with hyperkalaemia and trace quantities of calcium, have been studied and preliminary results are encouraging.

Apstein, Gravino & Haudenschild (1983) investigated the potential protective effects of glucose and insulin on ischaemic myocardium in rabbits and concluded that this combination affords protection during the period when glycogen has been depleted and when the myocardium is dependent on glucose as glycolytic substrate; glucose administered on its own has no beneficial effect. In contrast, Agakawa *et al.* (1983) found no significant advantage in adding glucose and insulin to a cold cardioplegic solution.

Other additives have also been studied. Many cardioplegic solutions, including the St Thomas and Bretschneider solutions, contain procaine probably on account of its membrane-stabilising effect. However, many units especially in the United States do not favour the inclusion of procaine. Ruigrok *et al.* (1985) found that the addition of thiopental has no effect on the appearance of ultrastructural damage during total ischaemia though it may afford some protection during low-grade ischaemia. Nayler, Gran & Yepez (1978) found that β-adrenoceptor antagonists such as verapamil and propranolol afford some protection to the myocardium. Slade & Nayler (1981) recorded that verapamil prevents lipid accumulation during ischaemic arrest and provides protection against reperfusion injury to myofibrillae and intercalated discs. Øskendal *et al.*

(1984) showed verapamil does afford protection to the myocardium but only if some traces of Ca^{2+} are present before perfusion. Other additives which have been tried include cortisone and glutamates (Kirklin & Barratt-Boyes, 1986).

The consensus of opinion suggests that a hyperkalaemic electrolyte solution can be successfully employed as a cardioplegic solution provided that it contains at least small quantities of Ca^{2+}. It should possess some buffering capacity and this may be provided by bicarbonate–carbonate, Tris or histidine buffers and osmotic pressure is maintained by an additive such as mannitol.

Coronary perfusion

When cardioplegia became temporarily unpopular about ten to twenty years ago, coronary perfusion was widely used for myocardial preservation. Fischer & Barner (1978), Nonoyama et al. (1978) and Shiraishi et al. (1980) investigated the effects of perfusion with cold oxygenated blood and concluded that it affords satisfactory protection for periods up to about 2.5 hours. Ferrans et al. (1972) observed that perfusion with filtered plasma does not prevent mitochondrial damage, extracellular oedema and swelling of SR; however, if the osmolarity of the plasma has been suitably adjusted by additives such as dextran, oedema is reduced and structural preservation is improved.

When electrolyte solutions are used for perfusion, oxygenation helps to maintain ATP and CP levels and mitochondrial respiratory activity above the critical level for over six hours and thus permits satisfactory resuscitation of the myocardium (Watanabe et al., 1978) and it also improves the prospects of functional and ultrastructural recovery during reperfusion.

Despite the results reported above, coronary perfusion fell into disfavour partly because its advantages were offset by reduction in the operating field. Moreover, artificial perfusion did not seem sufficiently effective for maintaining regions of subendocardial myocardium and damage to the coronary vasculature was also reported.

In regard to hearts removed for transplantation, Menz et al.

(1984) compared the effects of 24-h immersion storage with those of perfusion using a modified Krebs solution and found that myocardial ultrastructure preserved by either method showed little or no damage apart from minor blebbing of mitochondria; indeed the preservation in perfused specimens was less effective in that there was more mitochondrial swelling under such circumstances.

Effects of reperfusion

Reperfusion with blood after a limited period of cardiac arrest is able to reverse many of the ultrastructural changes caused by ischaemia in myocardial cells (Kloner et al., 1981; Schaper, Pinkowski & Froede, 1982; De Boer et al., 1983; Edonte et al., 1983; Goldstein & Murphy, 1983). As described in the earlier discussion, the critical duration before changes become irreversible is dependent on the circumstances. Under normothermic conditions without cardioplegia or coronary perfusion, irreversible changes probably set in within an hour but the critical interval can be extended for several hours by suitable protective manoeuvres. Further improvement occurs as reperfusion continues (Ashraf, Franklin & Nimmo, 1978; Lindal et al., 1983) but the sub-endocardial layers are less amenable to recovery than others probably because they are more resistant to reflow (Sunamori et al., 1978).

Although there is a general improvement of myocardial ultrastructure and function during reperfusion it is clear that, if no calcium is provided during the ischaemic phase, normal restoration of flow causes exacerbation of damage. The most striking features are contractile bands and pulling apart of cell membranes at the intercalated discs (Ashraf, White & Bloor, 1978; Boink, Ruigrok, Maas & Zimmerman, 1978; Totok, Trombitás & Röth, 1983; Humphrey, Thomson & Gavin, 1984; Ganote, 1986). There is substantial evidence that it is the restoration of calcium after a period of calcium deprivation that is responsible for the damage, although Humphrey & Vanderwee (1986) suggest that restoration of oxygen also plays a part. The role of calcium restoration (calcium paradox) was first identified by Zimmerman & Hülsman (1966) and it has been supported by evidence that reperfusion with calcium-free plasma preserves morphology better than calcium-containing media and that inclusion of a calmodulin inhibitor in the reperfusion medium also protects against damage (Schaffer, Burton, Jones & Oei, 1983). As pointed out earlier, reperfusion damage can be circumvented by providing small quantities of Ca^{2+} in the arrest phase (Jynge et al., 1978; Frank et al., 1983). The provision of verapamil in the arrest phase also seems to protect the myocardium against damage attributable to the calcium paradox (Slade & Nayler, 1981; Øskendal et al., 1984).

———

Insoluble triglycerides coalesce in the cytosol and appear in electron micrographs of cardiac myocytes as round, electron-lucent droplets without a limiting membrane. Comparative studies show that they are much more frequent in the myocardium of flying species such as the bat and of hibernating species like the hamster than of typical terrestrial mammals such as the rat and mouse. In all species, ventricular myocytes have a much higher content of lipid droplets than atrial myocytes.

All regions of the myocardium, including the nodal and conducting systems, have a high content of glycogen mainly in the form of smooth and ovoid β-granules. Myocardial glycogen is capable of providing about 1% of the energy requirements at rest and it becomes significantly depleted when the oxygen supply or blood supply to the heart wall is cut off.

Other effects of ischaemic arrest involve swelling of mitochondria with loss of function, reduction in high energy phosphates, changes in sarcolemmal ultrastructure and permeability, increase in lipid droplet number, margination of nuclear chromatin as well as cytosolic and extracellular oedema. Some changes are reversible up to about one hour after which they become permanent and more severe damage, including damage to myofibrillae, may set in. Protection against ischaemic damage can be afforded by cooling and by using high-potassium cardioplegic solutions to stop the heart in diastole; both techniques are employed for open heart surgery and for transplantation procedures. It is important to provide some Ca^{2+} during the arrest phase in order to avoid severe damage, such as contracture of myocytes and disruption of intercalated discs, which could occur when calcium is restored during reperfusion after a period of calcium starvation.

6

Atrial specific granules

Membrane-bound granules in the cytoplasm of cardiac myocytes were first described by Kisch (1956) and their presence has been confirmed repeatedly by numerous authors including Palade (1961), Jamieson & Palade (1964), Cantin & Huet (1975) and Navaratnam (1978). However, it has been only relatively recently that justifiable ideas regarding their composition and functions have emerged (see De Wardener & Clarkson, 1985; Lang *et al.*, 1985; Ballermann & Brenner, 1986; De Bold, 1986). They resemble the secretory granules of many endocrine glands and because, in mammals at least they are principally confined to atrial musculature, they have been termed atrial specific granules. However, they are not entirely exclusive to atrial myocytes; in lower vertebrates they are regularly found in ventricular cells and they may be occasionally encountered even in the mammalian ventricular wall (Kisch, 1963*a*; Rossi & Bassi, 1962) especially in neonatal or late foetal material. Nor are these granules uniformly distributed throughout the atrial musculature. Most accounts comment on their absence in the specialised slender cells of the sinu-atrial and atrioventricular nodes (Cheng, 1971; James *et al.*, 1966; Hayashi, 1971; Virágh & Porte, 1973*a,b*; Navaratnam, 1978, 1980) though Melax & Leeson (1970) describe their presence in the sinu-atrial node of the rat, Colborn & Garsey (1972) in the sinu-atrial node of the squirrel monkey and Bompiani, Rouiller & Hatt (1959) in the atrioventricular bundle of the rat. Granules are usually found in the working atrial myocardium especially that of the auricular appendages.

Some observers have claimed that different regions of atrial regions of atrial myocardium vary in granule density; for example Cantin *et al.* (1979) and McKenzie *et al.* (1985) claim that right atrial myocytes in the rat contain 2–2.5 times the number of granules in left atrial myocytes and Chapeau *et al.* (1985) describe a higher content in subepicardial muscle compared to deeper layers or the inter-atrial septum. However, in contrast with their findings in the rat, Cantin *et al.* (1979) reported that left atrial granule density in the guinea-pig greatly exceeds that of the right atrium whereas in several other species including the mouse and the hamster there is little or no difference. Comparative studies indicate also that atrial granules are largest and most numerous in small mammals such as the rat and the mouse, less so in the rabbit, guinea-pig and hamster and least in larger mammals including cat, dog, pig and man (Jamieson & Palade, 1964; Chapeau *et al.*, 1985). In general terms, therefore, there is an approximately inverse relationship between species size and atrial granularity though the golden hamster provides a striking exception (Figs. 6.1, 6.2); the fractional volume of granules in this species (0.0027) is less than one-tenth that in rats (0.028).

Ultrastructural appearance and distribution of atrial granules

In typical atrial myocytes, membrane-bound granules are most prevalent in the sarcoplasmic cone adjacent to the nuclear poles but they are also scattered among mitochondria in the columns between myofibrillae and some are situated subjacent to the sarcolemma (Figs. 2.8, 6.1). They are more or less spherical and the majority have a diameter of 200–400 nm with a range of about 100 to 500 nm depending on the species. Their contents are electron-dense and osmiophilic but a fine electron-lucent halo can often be discerned between the dense core and the limiting membrane. Many of the granules lie near Golgi elements, within the cisterns of which material of similar size and density may occasionally be found indicating that the granules are derived from the Golgi apparatus. Primary lysosomes containing dense material also bud off the Golgi apparatus but they can be distinguished from atrial granules by their smaller size (100–200 nm) and by their positive staining for acid phosphatase (see Fig. 6.3 and Chapter 7). Lipofuscin granules are scattered among atrial granules near the nuclear poles but they are distinguishable by their larger size and less-regular contour and, in some instances, by the retention of disrupted cristae in the matrix.

Some observers have classified atrial granules on the basis of their ultrastructural appearance and three categories have been described (see Cantin *et al.*, 1979): A-granules containing an intensely dense core, which is often eccentrically orientated and separated from the membrane by a distinctly clear gap (Fig. 6.4). B-granules which possess a paler fibrogranular core surrounded by a thin lucent halo; this variety appears to be less numerous. D-granules which are smaller in size than the others and resemble the characteristic granular vesicle of monoaminergic nerve varicosities. Of these, the existence of D-granules is questionable since they can be simulated by primary lysosomes in material not histochemically stained for acid phosphatase or by eccentric cuts through A- or B-granules. It is possible that the enhanced density and eccentrically placed contents of A-granules indicate a more mature and distended state than B-granules and that they are likely to be discharged earlier from the cell. Immunocytochemical labelling using antiserum to atriopeptin 28 and visualised by incubation with a secondary antibody conjugated with colloidal gold indicates that all granules are labelled and that A- and B-granules do not form distinct sets (Fig. 6.5). However, there is variation in the intensity of labelling which tends to increase proportionately with the electron density of the granule core.

In the adult, peripheral granules related to the sarcolemma are most frequent at those surfaces of atrial myocytes which lie near capillaries or atrial endocardium. This preferential distribution

Fig. 6.1. Electron micrograph of left atrial myocyte in an adult rat to show specific granules.

Fig. 6.2. Left atrial myocyte of adult golden hamster to show that the specific granules (g) are smaller and less numerous than those in the rat.

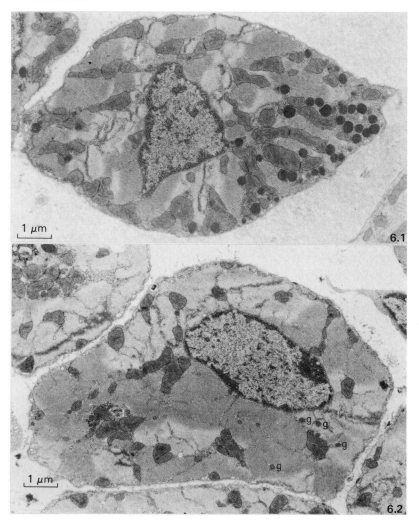

suggests that granule contents are released into the extracellular space and then transported across vascular endothelium into the circulation. The mechanism is almost certainly one of exocytosis, evidence for which is present in the form of 5-layered membrane images, where granules come in contact with the sarcolemma, and of occasional breaches in the membrane (Fig. 6.6). There is supporting evidence in freeze-fracture replicas where occasional granules are found bulging through the sarcolemma (Fig. 6.7) and *en face* views of the latter also show likely sites of exocytosis distinct from caveolae and T-tubules. The occurrence of granule discharge without manipulations of fluid or electrolyte balance indicates that there is a tonic level of release.

On the other hand, Theron, Biagio, Meyer & Boekkoi (1978) did not find evidence of exocytosis and suggested that granule contents are released into the cytoplasm. An alternative possibility to exocytosis is 'budding' of slender myocyte processes containing electron-dense material which may become detached from the parent cell. However, the irregular contour of the dense contents and the occasional retention of distorted cristae indicates that many of these buds contain lipofuscin material which remains unlabelled in immunocytochemical material. In terms of membrane economy, it is far more likely that waste material rather than granule secretion is discharged by the budding mechanism.

In several species including rats, mice and hamsters, the granules

Fig. 6.3. Rat atrial myocytes stained for acid phosphatase activity. Atrial specific granules (g), which are unstained for acid phosphatase, are larger than primary lysosomes (L_1) which are heavily stained for the enzyme. The granules are distributed both deeply and peripherally in the cytoplasm under tonic conditions.

Fig. 6.4. Rat atrial myocyte showing specific granules of the A and B varieties. Note the primary lysosomes (L_1) heavily stained for acid phosphatase.

Fig. 6.5. Rat atrial myocyte labelled with antibody to atriopeptin 28 conjugated with colloidal gold. Both A- and B-granules are labelled, though the labelling is heavier in the A-granules.

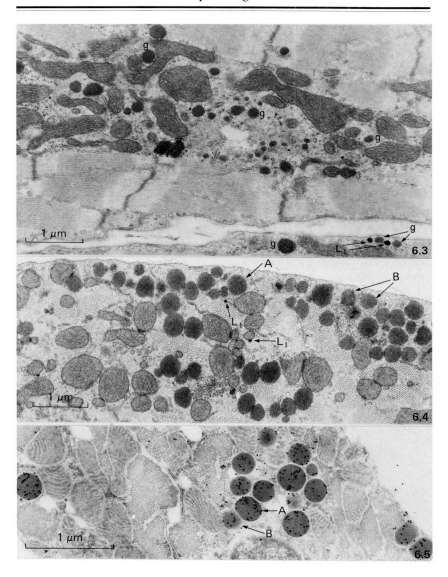

first appear in late foetal life just before birth. In human foetuses they are found during the fourth month of gestation (Fig. 6.8). They arise in the vicinity of the Golgi apparatus in both atrial and ventricular myocytes and initially they are few, not more than five in a single cell profile, and their contents are paler than in definitive granules. By the neonatal stage, the number of granules in atrial myocytes has increased strikingly whereas they are rare in ventricular cells. By the end of the first week of postnatal life, granules are practically undetectable in ventricular muscle whereas their distribution in atrial muscle has increased to levels similar to that in the adult.

Composition and functions of atrial granules

Till the mid-seventies, little was known about the composition of atrial granules apart from the presence of ATPase and other nucleotide phosphatase activity. Palade (1961) and Sosa-Lucero *et al.* (1969) had earlier suggested that atrial granules contain catecholamines on the grounds that (a) they resemble granules in the adrenal medulla, (b) extensive though incomplete degranula-

Fig. 6.6. Thin-section electron micrograph of rat atrial myocyte to show exocytosis of granule contents (arrow) under tonic conditions.

Fig. 6.7. Freeze-fracture replica of rat atrial myocyte to show a specific granule (g) bulging the surface sarcolemma prior to exocytosis.

Fig. 6.8. Thin section of atrial myocyte in a 4-month human foetus (90 mm C.R.) showing immature specific granules near the Golgi apparatus.

Fig. 6.9. Rat atrial myocardium 5 min after intravenous saline infusion showing accumulation of specific granules at a myocyte surface near the endocardial lumen (E).

Fig. 6.10. Rat atrial myocardium 5 min after intravenous saline infusion, the material having been labelled with antibody to atriopeptin 28 conjugated with colloidal gold. Immunoreactive granules show peripheralisation, near the sarcolemma, under these conditions.

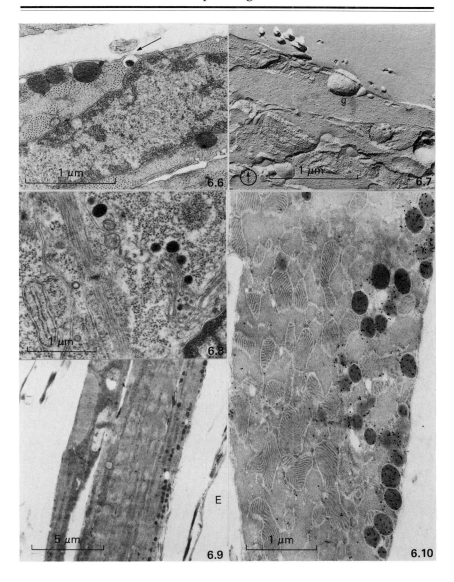

tion by reserpine administration had been reported (Palade, 1961), and (c) there is a mechanism for uptake of noradrenalin in heart muscle. Otsuka, Okamoto & Tomisawa (1969) and Tomisawa (1969) supported this view and reported that the density of staining could be enhanced by L-DOPA administration. However, other authors have not been able to confirm the degranulating effect of reserpine (Kisch, 1963b; Hibbs & Ferrans, 1969; De Bold & Bencosme, 1973; Yamauchi, 1973; Kuhn, Richards & Tranzer, 1975) and the granules have been found to be unaffected by the uptake of noradrenalin (Kuhn, Richards & Tranzer, 1975) or 5-hydroxydopamine. Moreover, atrial granules are not positive for histochemical tests for catecholamines and there is little correlation between regional granule content and catecholamine levels. Other possible functions considered for atrial granules included calcium storage (Blaineau-Peyretti & Nicaise, 1976) on the basis of ultrastructural studies of localisation of exogenously administered strontium but this view also failed to find support.

On the other hand, it has been shown conclusively that atrial granules lose electron density when treated with proteases such as pronase, trypsin or pepsin thus suggesting a substantial polypeptide content (Huet & Cantin, 1974b; Kuhn, Richards & Tranzer, 1975). This interpretation was strengthened by the finding that radioactively labelled amino acids are rapidly incorporated into atrial granules. Huet & Cantin (1974a) also showed that the granules contain carbohydrate complexes since they can be stained by methods such as the periodic thiocarbohydrazide-silver protein-ate technique or with phosphotungstic acid.

De Bold, Borenstein, Veress & Sonnenberg (1981) and Garcia et al. (1982) demonstrated that injection of homogenised atrial extract causes diuresis and natriuresis and that granule-rich fractions have the most potent effect. They postulated that the active principle, which can be termed atrial natriuretic factor (ANF) or atriopeptin, resides in the granules. In keeping with the comparative density and distribution of granules in different species, less natriuretic activity can be extracted from the atria of larger mammals and, in lower vertebrates, activity is found not only in atrial

muscle but also in the ventricles to a modest degree. Veress &
Sonnenberg (1984) showed that removal of the right auricular
appendix in the rat reduces renal responses to hypervolaemia and it
is now widely accepted that atrial granules can play a role in
electrolyte and fluid balance though some authorities have provided
dissenting evidence (see Knapp, Hicks, Linden & Mary, 1986).

In rat heart muscle the precursor of ANF is synthesised as a 152
amino acid preprohormone (151 in human). Cleavage of a 24
amino acid signal sequence and two other arginine residues leaves a
high molecular weight precursor, atriopeptigen, which can be
isolated from atrial extracts. A number of smaller biologically
active peptides also have been isolated from the atria and from
plasma of which the predominant circulating form is a 28 amino
acid cyclic peptide (3.06 kD) known as ser-leu-arg-arg atriopeptin
III or cardionatrin III (or simply as atriopeptin 28). Flynn, De Bold
& De Bold (1983) have established the primary structure of this
peptide in the rat as shown in the flow diagram below.

Kangawa & Matsuo (1984) subsequently reported the isolation,
sequencing and synthesis of a 28 amino acid peptide from human

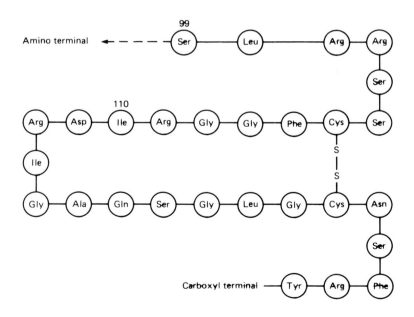

atria almost identical to that prepared from rat atria except that methionine occupies position 110 in the molecule instead of isoleucine. Most of the ANF-like material in atrial extracts is not identical to the plasma peptide; it probably represents a precursor and the conversion is believed to occur in the plasma. The identity of the active segment has not yet been determined, but, judging by the reactions of antisera to various fragments, it includes the 17 amino acid ring with the crucial disulphide bond to which extensions of variable length may be attached to the N- and C-terminals (Standaert, Saper & Needleman, 1985; Needleman, 1986).

The ANF gene from certain species including man has been sequenced and cloned so that various types of ANF can be produced by inserting the gene into bacteria or yeast or they can be synthesised. Antibodies have been raised against different forms of ANF, usually in the 21–28 amino acid sequence range, and have enabled scientists to study the localisation of ANF and to identify the sites where it is active, as well as to test the cross-reactivity of ANF antibody in different species, by means of immunochemical investigations at the light microscope and electron microscope levels (see Chapeau et al., 1985; McKenzie et al., 1985). Immunocytochemical techniques using HRP or colloidal gold labelling enable ANF-containing granules to be distinguished conclusively from neighbouring lysosomes and lipofuscin bodies. Radioimmunoassay techniques have enabled investigators to assess atriopeptin concentrations in atrial muscle and in the circulation (see Lang et al., 1985) and to monitor its release in response to experimental manoeuvres. Results in this laboratory indicate that the concentrations of immunoreactive atriopeptin 28 in unanaesthetised rats are as follows: left atrium, $157 \pm 22 \, \text{pmol mg}^{-1}$ wet tissue; right atrium, $180 \pm 26 \, \text{pmol mg}^{-1}$ wet tissue; plasma, $65 \pm 9.7 \, \text{fmol ml}^{-1}$ (Table 6.1); there is no significant difference between peptide concentrations in the two atria. These figures are higher than those reported by Lang et al. (1985), but similar to those of Takayanagi, Tanaka, Maki & Inagami (1985).

ANF has been shown to bind to receptor sites in the kidneys, adrenals, vascular smooth muscle and particular regions of the brain. It is believed to bring about its natriuretic and diuretic effects by a combination of complementary actions (Cantin & Genest, 1986) which include the following: (i) It reduces the secretion of renin thus inhibiting the effects of the renin-angiotensin mechanism. This in turn leads to reduced production of aldosterone and posterior pituitary vasopressin. (ii) It acts directly on the adrenal cortex inhibiting the secretion of aldosterone. (iii) ANF acts on the epithelial cells of kidney glomeruli and on related blood vessels, allowing larger quantities of water and sodium to be filtered from the blood; it also acts on tubules at the thin loop and distal tubule levels reducing the reabsorption of sodium. (iv) It acts on hypothalamic neurosecretory cells and their terminals in the pituitary, reducing the production and release of vasopressin. (v) ANF has a widespread vasodilator effect, most profoundly manifested by small vessels in the kidney, which complements other effects of ANF. Relaxation of vascular smooth muscle is probably mediated by activating cyclic GMP which affects Ca^{2+} entry or its cytoplasmic location. (vi) It binds to sites in the ciliary body possibly affecting the turnover of aqueous humor. (vii) It binds to the subfornical organ in addition to certain other sites in the brain (see p. 136).

In view of the numerous inter-related factors involved, it is extremely difficult to unravel the precise role played by release of ANF from the heart in maintaining fluid and electrolyte balance. Nevertheless, there is substantial experimental evidence to indicate that plasma levels of ANF are elevated when the circulation is loaded with fluid or salt and it is necessary to consider the possible underlying mechanisms.

Release of ANF in response to circulatory volume expansion

In a perceptive article, Smith (1957) suggested that there could be a circulating substance other than aldosterone that controls sodium secretion. Smith himself favoured the hypothalamus (see also Bealer *et al.*, 1983) as the likely site of production of this putative factor while other organs including the liver (Perlmutt, Aziz & Haberich, 1975) have also been suggested. Nevertheless, during the seventies, there were pointers that the atrial wall should be carefully investigated in this regard. Several investigators demonstrated that atrial distension causes an increase in urine flow and sodium excretion; most of the evidence arises from experiments causing distension of the left atrium (Carswell, Hainsworth & Ledsome, 1970; Gauer & Henry, 1976; Kappagoda et al., 1976), which seems to be more important in the control of water excretion, but Kappagoda, Linden & Snow (1973) did elicit a natriuretic response by increasing right atrial pressure. The diuretic effect of left atrial distension was thought to be due largely to vagally mediated inhibition of vasopressin secretion but Carswell and his colleagues showed, by cross-circulation experiments to an isolated kidney, that a humoral mechanism is also involved. These and other strands of evidence strongly indicated the existence of a hitherto unidentified hormone which could explain the concomitant occurrence of natriuresis and diuresis, a combination not accounted for by previously known regulatory factors. Keynes et al. (1982) observed a dissociation in the orthodox renin–aldosterone relationship in human subjects exposed to prolonged hypoxia at high altitude and they postulated the existence of an unknown factor.

It has become clear that increase in intravascular volume (Lang et al., 1985) or the administration of pressor agents (Manning et al., 1985) causes a 'dose-dependent' surge of ANF release into the circulation within one minute. Lang and his colleagues found that the mean plasma concentration of ANF in barbiturate-anaesthetised rats was $54.6 \pm 13.9 \, \text{pg} \, \text{ml}^{-1}$ (i.e. $17.8 \pm 4.5 \, \text{fmol} \, \text{ml}^{-1}$) and that infusion of 2 ml normal saline (corresponding to about 10% volume expansion and eliciting a 1–1.5-mm Hg peak in right atrial pressure) caused a 2–3-fold increase in plasma ANF concentration whereas administration of 8 ml saline (corresponding to about 30% volume expansion and eliciting a 5-mm Hg peak in atrial pressure) caused a 6-fold increase in ANF. The main form of circulating peptide is atriopeptin 28 but a quantity of precursor peptide is also secreted. Injection of ANF into hypertensive rats causes a significant but short-lived reduction of blood pressure and, in a line of rats genetically predisposed to hypertension, Cantin &

Genest (1986) found a high level of circulating ANF, probably an attempt by the body to reduce pressure. In hamsters prone to congestive cardiac failure, changes in ANF levels can be correlated with progress of the disease. Such findings indicate that, in these species at least, ANF is an important factor in maintaining circulatory homeostasis. In a recent article Anderson, Donckier, McKenna & Bloom (1986) report that intravenous infusions of saline in man significantly increase the circulating concentration of ANF without changes in plasma osmolality or electrolyte concentration from which they affirm that ANF is a circulating natriuretic factor and that atrial distension is an important stimulus for its release. Moreover, it has been demonstrated that the atrial muscle concentration of messenger RNA for ANF becomes depleted in response to water deprivation or volume depletion (Takayanagi et al., 1985; Zisfein et al., 1986) showing that the synthetic mechanism is sensitive to changes in blood volume. On the other hand, Knapp et al. (1986) claim that there is no evidence of natriuresis after atrial distension in vagotomised dogs although plasma levels of ANF are elevated, suggesting that ANF is causally unrelated to the normal natriuretic response.

Although the atrial wall is the most likely source of atriopeptin release on volume loading, this has not been definitely established. Experiments on rats in this laboratory show that intravenous infusion of 5 ml physiological saline, while causing an almost 4-fold increase in plasma atriopeptin level within 5 min, does not appear to affect the peptide concentration of atrial musculature which remains within control limits for both atria (Table 6.1); however, it should be pointed out that the atrial content (approximately 150–180 pmol mg^{-1} wet tissue, i.e. about 15 nmol/animal) is relatively massive compared to plasma levels (approximately 65 fmol ml^{-1}, i.e. about 650 fmol/animal) and may not show depletion unless there is protracted release. Moreover, morphometric studies do not indicate an alteration in the proportional volume occupied by granules in auricular myocytes; this remains steady at about 0.028 ± 0.004. Nevertheless, when granules situated within 1 μm of a sarcolemmal surface are enumerated, it is found that there is an increase of peripheral granules from approximately 32% in controls to over 50% in volume-loaded animals, confirming that there is a response to volume loading by the granules (Figs. 6.9, 6.10). The perinuclear population is correspondingly depleted. These findings contrast to some extent, though the experiments are not strictly comparable, with those of De Bold (1979) who found hypergranulation after water and salt deprivation, whereas the combined administration of deoxycorticosterone and 2% saline in drinking water leads to depletion of granules. In the same context, Thibault, Garcia, Cantin & Genest (1983) recorded that water deprivation is associated with increase in atrial granularity but with a significant decrease in acid-extractable natriuretic activity thus showing that the relationship between granule counts and atriopeptin content is not straightforward.

The exact mechanism involved in the release of ANF into the bloodstream is not clear but the persistence of ANF secretion in isolated perfused heart preparations indicates that direct stretch of atrial myocytes could be a key factor. It is uncertain whether, in addition, neuronal reflex arcs and brain centres are involved in the process (see Sonnenberg, 1985, for review). The experimental evidence concerning neuronal mediation in natriuresis is equivocal and, even if it does occur, there is no certainty that the neuronal link involves ANF release rather than another of the numerous factors

Table 6.1 *Radioimmunoassay values of atriopeptin concentration in atrial muscle and plasma in control and volume-loaded rats*

Schedule	Left atrium (pmol/mg wet tissue)	Right atrium (pmol/mg wet tissue)	Plasma (fmol/ml)
(a) Control	157 ± 22	180 ± 26	65.1 ± 9.7
(b) Volume-loaded (5 min after I.V. infusion of 5 ml physiological saline)	120 ± 12	141 ± 4	239.5 ± 52.5
(c) Sham-loaded	135 ± 12	128 ± 9	119.5 ± 22.0

Six adult animals in each group $\bar{x} \pm$ s.e.

known to affect salt and water balance; indeed, the evidence provided by Knapp *et al.* (1986) suggests that it is not. However, Gilmore & Daggett (1966) reported that total cardiac denervation in the dog reduces the renal response to dextran infusion, while Peterson, Felts & Chase (1983) reported similar results after dorsal root secretion and vagotomy-sinuaortic denervation in the monkey. Pearce & Sonnenberg (1965) found that natriuresis induced by an infusion of artificial blood in dogs with denervated kidneys is unaffected by bilateral vagotomy and they went on to report that it is completely abolished by spinal cord section at C8 level; other investigators, however, disagree with the interpretation that the afferent path for reflex natriuresis travels along the spinal cord (Bengele, 1971). Fater *et al.* (1982) reported that natriuresis induced by increasing left atrial pressure is eliminated by surgical intrapericardial denervation and they proposed that the afferent limb of the reflex arises very near the left atrium or in the right ventricle but not in the pulmonary bed. A consistent explanation of these and other experimental results does not seem possible, illustrating how difficult it is to make firm conclusions about each separate mechanism involved in salt and water balance.

The crucial question is whether changes in plasma ANF levels in various experiments are causally related to the renal elimination of sodium and water in the proportion required for volume correction. Balfour (1985) points out that the wide variation in the reported potency of the peptide is probably related to whether the animals are conscious or unconscious, hydrated or dehydrated, sodium deficient or replete.

ANF-like material in the brain

It is intriguing to find atriopeptin-like material in several distinct regions of the brain including areas of the hypothalamus, midbrain and hindbrain including the nucleus solitarius. The structure of the peptide in the brain has not yet been directly determined but radioimmunoassay, chromatography and molecular sizing of hypothalamic extracts strongly indicate that it is identical to the peptide found in the heart (Standaert, Saper & Needleman, 1985).

The most prominent group of atriopeptin immunoreactive neurons is found in the AV3V region of the hypothalamus near the anteroventral corner of the third ventricle. These neurons project to all divisions of the paraventricular nucleus as well as to regions concerned with cardiovascular and other autonomic regulation. Injection of ANF into the third ventricle suppresses vasopressin release and thus inhibits fluid intake; the effect is thought to be mediated at posterior pituitary and hypothalamic levels.

The nucleus solitarius is the point of relay for many of the primary afferents from the cardiovascular system and it includes the site of the baroreceptor reflex. Atriopeptin immunoreactive neurons are found in the medial part of the nucleus which is the region that receives most of the cardiovascular input. Similarly immunoreactive neurons are also found in the parabrachial nucleus and in other regions such as the ventrolateral medulla both of which are relay sites for nucleus solitarius projections. In addition, reactive neurons are found in parts of the limbic system including the habenular, mammillary and dorsal tegmental nuclei. Using peptides labelled with radioactive iodine, specific ANF-binding sites have been found in the septal region and subfornical organ in addition to parts of the hypothalamus.

The distribution of atriopeptin within the CNS in precisely those regions which are concerned in the regulation of fluid and electrolyte balance and of the cardiovascular system, is unlikely to be an irrelevant coincidence. The significance of such reciprocity between peripheral and brain peptides (other examples include cholecystokynin and angiotensin) is still unclear but it is possible that atriopeptin-sensitive neurons in the brain provide a mechanism for recognition of ANF levels in the blood or the cerebrospinal fluid or both, and could operate by co-ordinating the relevant homeostatic mechanisms; the possibility that atriopeptin acts as a neurotransmitter or as a neuromodulator in the brain has also been suggested (Standaert, Saper & Needleman, 1985).

The idea that there is a natriuretic hormone released by the brain was initiated by Smith (1957) and more recently supported by the experiments of Bealer et al. (1983), who found that plasma from volume-expanded rats contains an agent which inhibits sodium transport in toad bladders but that volume-expanded rats with AV3V lesions lack this plasma agent. Bealer and his colleagues argued that either the agent is produced by the AV3V region in response to raised [Na$^+$] or that the AV3V is crucial in causing the release of a natriuretic agent from another site. Although there seems to be a reasonable consensus that sodium excretion is influenced by brain sodium concentration, the efferent mechanism is not clear. In any case, differential perfusion experiments show that the excretory effect of an increase of brain sodium concentration is probably fairly weak and cannot override sodium retention caused by pre-existing general sodium depletion.

Other possible sites of ANF synthesis

Using antiserum to a synthetic 25 amino acid sequence (atriopeptin IV), McKenzie *et al.* (1985), have reported immunoreactive sites in the salivary gland, renal collecting ducts, adrenal medullary chromaffin cells and gonadotrophs of the anterior pituitary in the rat. The list of such reactive sites is likely to expand, but there is little information on the physiological roles played by such widespread resources of ANF.

General atrial myocardial cells are characterised by the presence of numerous spherical, membrane-bound granules, possessing an osmiophilic core and measuring about 200–400 nm in diameter. They are rarely present in ventricular myocytes or in nodal cells. The contents of the granule are released into the bloodstream in response to increased circulatory volume or salt and have the effects of natriuresis, diuresis and vasodilation. The precursor of the active principle is synthesised as a 152 amino acid polypeptide and is stored in atrial granules. A number of smaller biologically active compounds also have been isolated from the atria and from plasma of which the commonest circulating form is a 28 amino acid cyclic peptide (atriopeptin 28).

Radioimmunoassay studies in control rats indicate that the concentration of immunoreactive atriopeptin 28 in atrial muscle is about $157-180\,\mathrm{pmol\,mg^{-1}}$ wet tissue (15 nmol/animal) and the plasma concentration is about $65\,\mathrm{fmol\,ml^{-1}}$ (650 fmol/animal) indicating tonic release. Intravenous infusion of 5 ml physiological saline causes an almost four-fold increase in plasma peptide content without affecting the larger atrial peptide level. Morphometric studies of material labelled with antibody to atriopeptin 28 conjugated with colloidal gold indicate that the proportional volume of atrial myocytes occupied by granules remains unchanged at about 0.028 but there is increased peripheralisation and exocytosis of granules.

7

Ultrastructural changes in ageing myocardial cells

There is no doubt that cardiac efficiency declines in old age. In humans, the functional capacity of the cardiovascular system has been estimated to decline continuously at the rate of approximately 1% each year beyond the age of 30 (see Goldberg, 1978, for review); heart rate and cardiac output appear to decrease with age whereas systemic blood pressure and peripheral resistance increase. Similar age-associated changes have been reported in rodents and Goldberg concluded from a study on rats that bradycardia in old age is caused by changes in the heart itself and in its noradrenergic innervation. Electrophysiological changes have been reported in both man and laboratory animals which may underlie the high incidence of dysrhythmic conditions in older individuals. Electrocardiographic alterations include prolongation of the P-R interval, QRS complex and the S-T segment. Experiments on animals have shown that there is decreased contractility, comprising both reduced velocity and amplitude of shortening, of the myocardium which consequently takes longer time to develop peak tension (Heller & Whitehorn, 1974); decrease in sinu-atrial node rate has also been reported (Cavoto, Kelleher & Roberts, 1974) resulting from alterations in transmembrane potential, decreased rate of rise in potential, increased plateau duration and increased re-polarisation time. Biochemical changes such as reduced myosin ATPase activity and decreases in protein content and protein synthesis have also been recorded.

Despite the well documented decline in cardiac function with advancing age, early investigators found it difficult to attribute the changes to biological age alone. Part of the difficulty arose from heavy reliance on human studies and many investigators inclined to the view expressed by Pomerance (1976) – 'Most of the findings generally regarded as typical of the elderly heart are not expressions of normal senescence, but of pathological processes that show increasing incidence with age'. The only structural change consistently noted in human myocardial cells was accumulation of lipofuscin, the origin and significance of which was unclear. However, in more recent times considerable advances in knowledge have resulted from the use of selected healthy animal colonies for laboratory studies on ageing where careful screening could be maintained against infection. In this manner, apart from observations on lipofuscin formation it has been possible to follow possible alterations in the ultrastructure of cardiac myocytes in regard to a variety of organelles including the sarcoplasmic reticulum, mitochondrial content (Herbener, 1976) and myofilament organisation (Feldman & Navaratnam, 1981).

Lipofuscin formation

As mammalian cardiac myocytes age, large numbers of electron-dense osmiophilic organelles accumulate within their cytoplasm (Fawcett & McNutt, 1969). These organelles have been termed variously, lipofuscin, dense bodies, age pigment and residual bodies and they are also found in certain other tissues such as neurons of the central and peripheral nervous systems (Peters, Palay & Webster, 1970), cells of the anterior pituitary (Smith & Farquhar, 1966), liver (Essner & Novikoff, 1960) and skeletal muscle (Fundoianu-Dayan, Abrahami, Buchner & Gorsky, 1985). The fractional volume of cardiac myocytes occupied by lipofuscin is substantial and some estimates, for instance those of Strehler, Mark, Mildban & Gee (1959) for the human heart, place it as high as 6% though other investigators believe this is an overestimate (Sachs, Colgan & Lazarus, 1977). The rate of accumulation is probably not uniform and the finding that lipofuscin formation in the hamster heart is slowed during hibernation (Lyman, O'Brien & Green, 1981; Papafrangas & Lyman, 1982) indicates that the process may be influenced by the work load of the myocardium.

Lipofuscin granules appear in the myocardium and other tissues early in development, for instance they are found in the rat and hamster myocardium by 2–3 months after birth (Feldman & Navaratnam, 1981; Skepper & Navaratnam, 1987) and, indeed, observations on mouse embryos suggest that their formation has commenced before birth. Nevertheless, the precise origin of these bodies is still unclear. Some authors have suggested a lysosomal origin (Samarajski, Ordy & Keeffe, 1965; Samarajski, Ordy & Rady-Reimer, 1968; Peters, Palay & Webster, 1970; Hasan & Glees, 1972) on the basis of ultrastructural studies. Their view is supported by other investigators employing histochemical techniques under the light microscope (Gedigk & Bontke, 1956; Goldfischer, Villaverde & Forschirm, 1966) and under the electron microscope (Essner & Novikoff, 1960, 1961; Frank & Christianson, 1968; Novikoff, Novikoff, Quintana & Hauw, 1971; Decker, 1974). On the other hand, biochemical studies of isolated lipofuscin have not shown lysosomal enzyme activity (Malkoff & Strehler, 1963; Hendley & Strehler, 1965). Other authors have suggested an exclusively or predominantly mitochondrial origin for lipofuscin bodies based on descriptions of standard ultrastructure (Feldman & Navaratnam, 1981; Koobs, Schultz & Jutzy, 1978; Sachs et al., 1977; Spoerri & Glees, 1973; Travis & Travis, 1972). Some of these authors indicated that other organelles such as lipid, glycogen and Golgi elements can also be degraded to form lipofuscin but to a lesser extent than mitochondria (Ghosh, Bern, Ghosh & Nishioka, 1962; Travis & Travis, 1972).

In studying the relationship between lipofuscin and lysosomes, acid phosphatase (AP) activity which is known to be a characteristic feature of lysosomes (De Duve, 1964; Goldfischer, 1982; Novikoff, 1963, 1964; Novikoff, Essner & Quintana, 1964) is a valuable marker. Although lysosomes are known to contain numerous hydrolytic enzymes including proteases, nucleases, phosphatases, glycosidases, lipases, phospholipases and sulphatases (see Butcher, 1983), AP is relatively specific to lysosomes and their precursors and it is conveniently demonstrable by histochemical techniques. The following descriptions are based on electron microscope studies of the myocardium of albino rats (2 months to 32 months), from an outbred Sprague-Dawley derived strain maintained as an ageing colony, and of golden hamsters (2 months to 18 months) of the WO strain. Some of the material was stained for AP activity by a lead-precipitation technique using sodium β-glycerophosphate as substrate (Lewis & Knight, 1977; modified from Barka & Anderson, 1962).

AP activity in Golgi apparatus and primary lysosomes

In atrial myocytes, the Golgi apparatus is found close to the nuclear membrane both at the poles and alongside the length of the nucleus. The cisternae at the maturing or *trans* face of the Golgi are intensely positive for AP and some of its positive elements are found in more peripheral situations. In ventricular myocytes, Golgi components are less extensive and the AP activity is less intense; nonetheless, they can be recognised both deep in the cytoplasm and near the periphery.

Lysosomes are not easy to identify on general ultrastructural features, particularly in the atrial myocardium where the specific granules are somewhat similar in shape and general appearance. Spherical membrane-bound granules measuring 100–200 nm in diameter can be seen budding off Golgi complexes in both atrial and ventricular myocardium. Sections studied after the AP reaction reveal that a high proportion of these organelles give a positive reaction thus confirming them as primary lysosomes and, when slightly thicker sections are examined, these AP-positive granules are found to be continuous with the region where the endoplasmic reticulum impinges on the Golgi apparatus; this region clearly constitutes the so-called GERL (Golgi–endoplasmic reticulum–lysosome) complex. Atrial specific granules, on the other hand, show no reaction for AP (Fig. 6.8) and they are usually larger. Despite their origin from the Golgi apparatus, primary lysosomes are not restricted to its vicinity and they assume no preferential localisation in the cytoplasm of either atrial or ventricular myocytes. The majority are near-spherical in shape but a small proportion are tubular.

Degradative changes in cardiac myocytes

The earliest and most frequently observed degradative changes are those associated with mitochondria. The evidence in mouse material shows that such changes are initiated even before birth and that they increase in frequency with age so that they are readily observed in atrial and ventricular myocytes in juvenile animals. The degenerating mitochondria appear to undergo a progressive condensation which can be detected even in material not stained for AP. At the simplest stage, there is increased electron density at the periphery and, to a lesser extent, in central foci within mitochondria. As degeneration progresses the cristae become altered or disappear and the matrix contains conspicuous osmiophilic material dispersed in several foci (Figs. 7.4, 7.5). These organelles are recognisable as mitochondria only because they retain the characteristic limiting double membrane and, in some instances, a laminar component can be discerned within the matrix; at high magnifications, these components often appear pentalaminar with dark margins and a lighter streak in which a central linear density is situated. Similar osmiophilic material, but lacking limiting membranes, is seen in the cytoplasm sometimes as a single clump but more often in small groups.

Even in material that has not been stained for AP activity there are indications that most degradative changes in mitochondria are associated with lysosomal activity. For instance, quite frequently, small organelles resembling primary lysosomes are found apposed to or in the close vicinity of mitochondria undergoing early condensation change. Histochemical staining for AP confirms that such organelles attached to mitochondria are indeed primary lysosomes (Figs. 7.1, 7.2). The target mitochondrion itself may show no AP activity initially as in Fig. 7.1 but, after lysosomal fusion, AP activity appears at the periphery (Fig. 7.2) and later at the centre corresponding to the foci of enhanced electron density. Such a body constitutes a form of secondary lysosome. Where the plane of section has not cut the primary lysosome, it is still possible to detect the effects of AP activity by viewing material not obscured by further metallic staining. In such preparations, even low concentrations of AP reaction product can be discerned (Fig. 7.3).

As the animals grow older, intensely osmiophilic but AP-negative bodies (lipofuscin) are found in addition to AP-positive secondary lysosomes of mitochondrial origin (Figs. 7.6, 7.7). Often the two types lie in the same field of view and their appearances can be compared; in some instances, especially in the atrial myocardium, it is possible to find several intermediary stages in the same myocyte. Figure 7.6, for example, demonstrates a primary lysosome with

Fig. 7.1. Atrial myocyte from a 3-month-old hamster stained for AP. The field includes an AP-positive primary lysosome attached to a mitochondrion which shows little structural change and contains no intrinsic AP activity.

Fig. 7.2. Atrial myocyte from a 4-month-old hamster stained for AP. The micrograph shows a primary lysosome attached to a degraded mitochondrion. The periphery of the mitochondrion is AP positive, like the lysosome, and its cristae are grossly distorted.

Fig. 7.3. Atrial myocyte from a 4-month-old hamster. The material was stained for AP but unosmicated and not stained further. Scattered AP activity is seen throughout the matrix of a degraded mitochondrion but the associated lysosome cannot be seen in this plane of section. Picture by courtesy of Mr J.N. Skepper.

Fig. 7.4. Atrial myocyte from a 3-month-old hamster unstained for AP. It contains a mitochondrion which shows degradative changes comprising enhanced osmiophilia especially at the periphery of the organelle and also at its centre. The cristae can be discerned in parts and the double limiting membrane is clearly seen.

Fig. 7.5. Mitochondrion in a ventricular myocyte from a 4-month-old hamster; material unstained for AP. The limiting membrane can be discerned but not the cristae. Patches of increased density are scattered throughout the matrix of the organelle.

Fig. 7.6. Atrial myocyte from a 5-month-old hamster stained for AP. The field includes a series of organelles including AP-positive primary lysosomes (L_1), secondary lysosomes (L_2) and a lipofuscin body (L_f) lacking AP. There are also several, specific atrial granules in the cell.

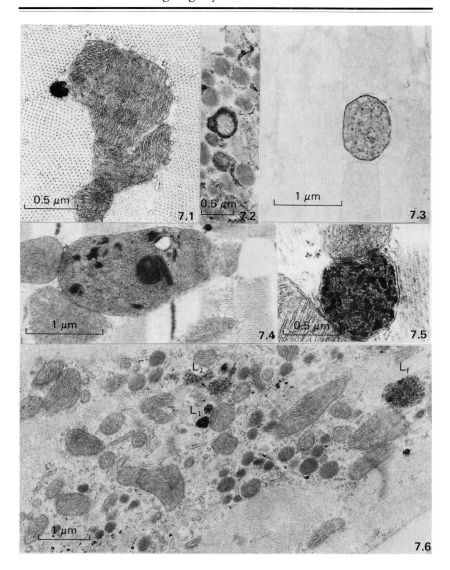

7.1

0.5 μm

7.2

0.5 μm

7.3

1 μm

7.4

1 μm

7.5

0.5 μm

7.6

1 μm

intense AP activity close to a mitochondrion, in addition to several secondary lysosomes with less-pronounced enzyme activity and an osmiophilic but AP-negative lipofuscin body. The sequence suggests that the lipofuscin granule is a terminal lysosome which has lost its AP activity.

In young animals dense-body profiles are round or oval, have smooth contours and are of similar size to mitochondria. With advancing age, however, irregularities of shape become more frequent and they enlarge appreciably so that in senile animals they can be several times the size of the largest mitochondrion. The increases in size and irregularity suggest that lipofuscin granule growth occurs by coalescence or accretion.

Dense bodies with globular components resembling those in neuronal lipofuscin do not appear in rat myocardium except in the oldest animals (31–32 months) and even then the globules are very small. In hamsters, on the other hand, globular bodies are present by 5–6 months and they become more conspicuous with age especially in ventricular myocytes (Figs. 7.8, 7.9). There is evidence to suggest that they are produced in a manner different to that described for the majority of dense bodies. In these older animals,

Fig. 7.7. Ventricular myocyte from a 6-month-old hamster stained for AP. The field includes an AP-positive secondary lysosome (L_2) which retains a smooth outline, and a larger AP negative lipofuscin body (L_f) which has an irregular outline and contains several foci of increased osmiophilia and a globule.

Fig. 7.8. Ventricular myocyte from a 6-month-old hamster unstained for AP. The field includes a clump of osmiophilic debris lacking a limiting membrane and a globular lipofuscin body possessing a membrane.

Fig. 7.9. Ventricular myocyte from a 6-month-old hamster unstained for acid phosphatase. The micrograph shows lipid droplets which are individually or collectively enclosed by a limiting membrane, presumably that of an autophagic vacuole. There is increased osmiophilia in parts of the organelle.

Fig. 7.10. Left atrial myocyte from an 18-month-old rat, showing a large mass of helically aggregated strands (asterisk) between fascicles of unaltered myofilaments. Note several atrial specific granules in the field.

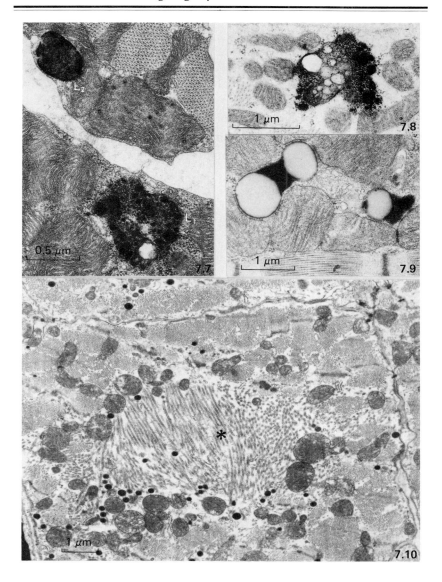

occasional autophagic vacuoles are found in both atrial and ventricular myocytes. Such vacuoles are bound by a limiting membrane and some contain the remnants of mitochondria. They possess moderate AP activity patchily distributed within the vacuole but the manner of their interaction with primary lysosomes is not clear. Other material which is degraded in comparable fashion includes lipid droplets and unidentifiable amorphous debris. Degenerating lipid droplets show a sharp increase in osmiophilia at the periphery and this is accompanied by the appearance of a limiting membrane, probably that of an autophagic vacuole; in many instances, more than one droplet is enclosed within the body. Material stained for AP shows enzyme activity coincident with the osmiophilic periphery confirming the incorporation of lysosomal activity. At more advanced stages, especially in bodies containing numerous small globules, staining for AP is absent.

The foregoing evidence suggests strongly that most or all lipofuscin granules are terminal lysosomes. Previous investigators including Glees (1985), Hasan & Glees (1972), Peters *et al.* (1970), Samarajski *et al.* (1965, 1968) and Tomanek & Karlsson (1972) postulated that lysosomes are involved in the production of lipofuscin without elucidating the manner of involvement. Travis & Travis (1972), in a description of rat ventricular myocytes based on standard ultrastructural material without enzyme histochemistry, argued that lipofuscin granules are formed by the action of lysosomal enzymes on organelles especially mitochondria and similar findings in neural tissue were reported by Holtzman, Novikoff & Villaverde (1967). In another study Cano, Hervas & Machado (1981) described myelin-like inclusions in maturing and senescent rat myocardium, some of which are closely applied to lipid droplets, and suggested that the figures are derived from lysosomes.

The most frequently observed sequence of degradation accords well with that suggested by Travis & Travis (1972); it comprises fusion of primary lysosomes, which bud off the GERL complex, with scattered mitochondria. After lysosomal fusion, the mitochondrial outer membrane remains intact but an increase in peripheral density occurs. Travis & Travis suggested that the increase in density is caused by the hydrolytic action of lysosomal enzymes and this view is supported by the finding that AP staining has a similar distribution to that of electron-dense foci. Moreover, Barka (1964) and Robinson & Karnovsky (1983) provided evidence that organelles undergoing degradation are initially attacked by hydrolytic enzymes at their periphery. According to Koobs *et al.* (1978), the increase in electron density can be ascribed to the byproduct malonaldehyde which causes the binding of unsaturated lipid to protein and nucleic acids leaving a highly osmiophilic residue. Although the enhancement of electron density starts peripherally, it subsequently spreads through the organelle. The organelle thus condenses through intermediate stages to form a terminal lysosome or lipofuscin body which retains a recognisable double membrane. AP activity persists through the intermediate stages in the matrix of the body, as has been described for other tissues by Essner & Novikoff (1961) and Frank & Christianson (1968), but it eventually becomes depleted; this is possibly another effect of malonaldehyde which is known to inactivate many groups of enzymes (Chio & Tappel, 1969).

Residual lipofuscin bodies can be visualised under the light microscope as a brown or yellow pigment which is autofluorescent. The elegant light microscope studies of Barden (1970) demonstrated a transformation with age of AP-positive non-fluorescent granules to AP-negative autofluorescent residual structures. When enzyme activity disappears, the organelle can be said to represent a terminal lysosome or lipofuscin granule. There is biochemical evidence to support this interpretation. For instance, Malkoff & Strehler (1963) isolated lipofuscin from the human heart and found it to be AP-negative and, in a subsequent study, Hendley & Strehler (1965) using density gradient centrifugation found AP activity in a more slowly sedimenting band than lipofuscin.

The predominantly mitochondrial origin of lipofuscin was supported by quantitative data which revealed a reduction of mitochondrial number with age (Herbener, 1976) and by observations that mitochondrial enzyme activity is also depleted (Abu-

Erreish & Sanadi, 1978). Moreover, Colcolough, Hack, Heleny, Vaugh & Veith (1972) isolated significant amounts of flavin, which is normally present in mitochondria, from lipofuscin. Mitochondrially derived lipofuscin bodies are smooth in outline and relatively small in size. Less common in young animals are the larger globular variety with an irregular outline. The findings suggest that such bodies arise in older members by the activity of autophagic vacuoles which engulf miscellaneous organelles including lipid droplets and mitochondria. They initially contain AP which eventually declines as in the commoner form. The ingestion of lipid droplets in particular follows a characteristic pattern leaving a number of electron-dense globules. A similar process of lipid droplet degradation coincident with changes in AP activity has been reported in neural tissue by Frank & Christianson (1968).

The reason that globular bodies are very rare in the rat heart compared to hamsters, except in senile animals (Feldman & Navaratnam, 1981), is possibly because cardiac myocytes in the rat possess relatively few lipid droplets. Even in the hamster, globular bodies are more frequent in ventricular myocytes where droplets are more prominent than in atrial myocardium (Navaratnam, Ayettey, Addae, Kesse & Skepper, 1986).

Most lipofuscin granules accumulate progressively within the myocyte cytoplasm mainly at two preferential sites. The first of these is along the columns of mitochondria which lie between myofibrillae. The second preferential site is within the sarcoplasmic cone at each nuclear pole where dense bodies are interspersed among mitochondria and lysosomes and, in atrial cells, specific granules. A very small number of lipofuscin granules have been observed while being extruded from myocytes into the intercellular space in small cell processes containing some cytoplasm and enclosed by sarcolemma (Skepper & Navaratnam, 1987). They are then probably engulfed by scavenger cells such as histiocytes or by capillary endothelium (Coleman, Silbermann, Gershon & Reznick, 1982). There is evidence to suggest that drugs such as centrophenoxine and lucidril reduce the lipofuscin content of neurons by accelerating their elimination (Spoerri & Glees, 1974) and it is possible that there are similar effects on cardiac myocytes.

Other mitochondrial changes

The degradation of mitochondria by lysosomal action into dense bodies or lipofuscin is only one of several ways to account for age-related deficits in mitochondrial number and activity. Other mitochondrial abnormalities have been observed in the cardiac myocytes of rats (Feldman & Navaratnam, 1981) and mice (Tate & Herbener, 1976) in which lysosomes do not appear to be implicated. These abnormalities include hypertrophy of mitochondria coupled with apparent disruption of the cristae, or even dissolution where the interior of the organelle consists of homogeneous matrix. Lysosomes have not been identified in the vicinity of such hypertrophied organelles and the lack of AP staining indicates that they are not involved, at least initially, in their genesis. Hypertrophic changes occur in individual scattered mitochondria, neighbouring organelles usually being unaffected. Such disruption is more prevalent in older animals but it has been seen occasionally in the juvenile group.

A second type of abnormality, also AP-negative but considerably more common than hypertrophy, seems to be confined to older animals especially those in the senile group. It consists of ensheathment of a mitochondrion by multiple lamellae closely applied to the mitochondrial surface. It has not yet proved possible to determine whether they are continuous or discrete. In some instances, however, the peripheral lamellae appear to be closely associated with cisterns of sarcoplasmic reticulum, suggesting that the reticulum may be involved in the synthesis of the sheath membrane. Travis & Travis (1972) considered the lamellae to be derived from autophagic vacuoles (secondary lysosomes) but the lack of AP activity renders this unlikely.

The mitochondria which are ensheathed might display a variety of intrinsic structural abnormalities, particularly disruption or dissolution of cristae. In addition, what appear to be remnants of sheaths containing degenerated material are occasionally encountered along mitochondrial rows between myofibrillae. These observations suggest that ensheathment followed by mitochondrial degeneration is a possible sequence in age-related loss of mitochondria. Thus there appears to be a range of sequences possible, some of which are dependent on lysosomal activity and others which are not. It is not clear whether both types of sequence lead to the formation of lipofuscin granules.

A further observation noticed only in old animals comprises the accumulation of large numbers of small mitochondria in sarcoplasmic tracts between myofibrillae. When examined under high magnification many of these mitochondria are found to exhibit abnormalities such as disruption of cristae or matrix vacuolisation.

Abnormal filamentous arrays

Unusual filamentous arrays in the form of helically aggregated strands appear in cardiac myocytes of young adult animals and increase in frequency as they age. For instance, in samples of right auricular appendage from rats more than 18 months old they could be found in every grid examined (Feldman & Navaratnam, 1981). Similar structures have been described by Leeson (1980) in the right atrial wall of 2–6-month-old rats and he suggested that their function might be related to 'the special conducting system known to exist in the right atrium'. However, systematic search does show that abnormal arrays are present in the musculature of all cardiac chambers in senile animals although they are more profuse in atrial muscle.

Typically in atrial muscle, the abnormal filamentous arrays lie in large clusters within the sarcoplasm (Fig. 7.10), occupying space that in other cells would be occupied by normal myofilaments, and they often extend across the full thickness of the cell. In addition there could be smaller foci of helically aggregated strands, situated between fascicles of normal myofilaments which are easy to over-look unless one specifically seeks them. Each strand is composed of what appear to be two or more elements or subunits wound round each other in helical fashion (Fig. 7.11). Where the orientation of the strand is parallel to the plane of section a strand can be resolved into two elements at some points along its course but more than two elements at other points. Preliminary measurements indicate that each element is about 12 nm thick (Leeson's measurements indicate a slightly finer filament 9–11 nm in diameter). In most, but not all, instances of helically aggregated strands cut longitudinally there is a fine transverse striation between the elements giving the appearance of cross-bridges; the distance between successive striations is 15–20 nm. In oblique sections (Figs. 7.11, 7.13) typically short, crescentic profiles are seen. While sometimes such profiles appear to be composed of only two filamentous elements, multiple stranding is more commonly suggested.

Figures 7.12 and 7.13 show some of these strands in cross-section and they reveal quadratic lattices or grids which contain several filaments (usually ranging between 6 and 16) interlinked by cross-bridges; the cross-bridges measure about 4–5 nm in thickness. In several instances, apparent transitions between normal fascicles of myofilaments and the helically aggregated strands are observed. When such a transitional zone is viewed in transverse section it gives the impression that individual thick myofilaments have separated from a normal fascicle to lie in rosette-like groups which frequently have five filaments. These aggregates then appear to undergo transition to the quadratic lattice form. Evidence of similar transition can be seen in the longitudinal plane where it appears that thick myofilaments have become rearranged from their normal pattern to form helically aggregated strands. The centre-to-centre separation of 12-nm filaments in a typical quadratic lattice is 25–30 nm (for comparison, the thick myofilaments at A-band level in a normal myofibril have a thickness of up to 15 nm; they are hexagonally arranged and their centre-to-centre separation is about 35–45 nm).

The chemical composition of the filaments comprising these curious arrays has not been entirely resolved but preliminary immunocytochemical studies as well as their ultrastructural configuration indicate that they are composed of a type of myosin aggregation. In many instances there is apparent continuity or transition between normally arranged thick filaments and the elements of the helical strands: indications of such transition can be observed both among filaments cut longitudinally and in those cut transversely. It is also worth noting that the cross-bridges between the strand filaments display a periodicity of 15–20 nm compared to a spacing of 14 nm found for cross-bridges in skeletal muscle. On the other hand, Leeson (1978) reports a spacing of 30 nm which contrasts sharply with these figures. The significance of helically aggregated strands is not known and it is not clear whether they represent the disruption of myofilaments which had previously been arranged in normal fashion or whether they arise *de novo* with advancing age. It does seem reasonable, however, to assume that their presence represents an impediment to the normal contractile behaviour of muscle cells; a normal mode of contraction would seem unlikely in view of their intertwining nature and the absence of thin filaments.

Other changes in cardiac myocytes

Other abnormal features noticeable in senile animals include patches of atypically expanded Z-line material. Such expanded patches are more frequently found near collections of helically aggregated strands and seem to be associated with poor anchoring of thin filaments. Similar expansion of electron-dense material is observed in relation to the intermediate junction segments of intercalated discs where thin filaments should normally be inserted. In addition, some degenerative foci comprising loose electron-dense material also appear in some myocytes in ageing animals. Like the

Fig. 7.11. Enlargement of Fig. 7.10 to show helically-aggregated strands. In longitudinal section, the strand composition varies from simple twining of elements to more complex arrangements. Cross-bridges can be seen in the strands indicated by arrows. Ob indicates the crescentic appearance of strands viewed in oblique section.

Fig. 7.12. Left atrial myocardium from a 6-month-old rat showing a myocyte with large numbers of abnormal strands cut in cross-section when they reveal a lattice-like arrangement.

Fig. 7.13. Another atrial myocyte from a 6-month-old rat showing abnormal strands in cross-section.

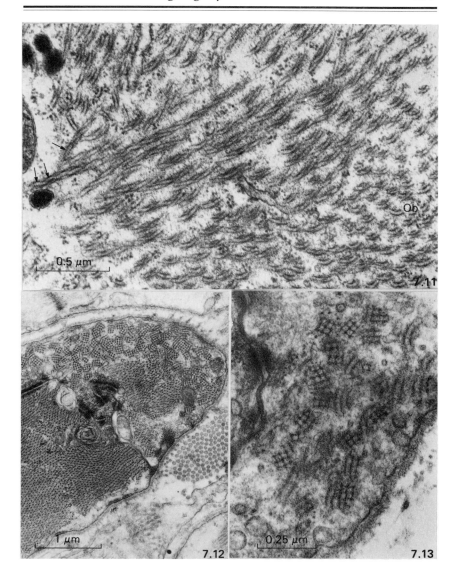

7.11

7.12

7.13

patches of expanded Z-line material, some of these foci lie near accumulations of helically aggregated strands.

Cells containing abnormal features such as helically aggregated strands, expanded Z-lines and degenerating foci are often characterised by an increase in nucleolar material. This suggests that there is enhanced RNA synthesis and possibly protein synthesis in such cells but there is little or no biochemical or histochemical information on this problem.

———

Lipofuscin formation begins very early in life and accelerates with advancing age. The main sequence in atrial and ventricular myocytes is by fusion of acid phosphatase (AP)-positive primary lysosomes with mitochondria, which are progressively degraded and the matrix becomes denser with an accompanying increase in AP activity. After reaching a peak level, AP activity declines until an AP-negative terminal pigment body with a smooth outline is produced. Another sequence leads to the formation of larger, irregular bodies containing small globules. Their genesis entails the participation of autophagic vacuoles which engulf lipid droplets or amorphous debris. Like the commoner variety of lipofuscin, they contain AP while digestion progresses but eventually become AP negative. Age-related changes not associated with lysosomal activity include mitochondrial hypertrophy with apparent disruption or even dissolution of cristae.

Unusual filamentous arrays in the form of helically aggregated strands appear in the sarcoplasm of young adult animals and increase in frequency with age. Immunocytochemical studies indicate that they may be composed of a type of myosin aggregation unassociated with thin filaments. Patches of expanded Z-line material may be found near helically aggregated strands and other abnormal features in senile animals include degenerative foci comprising loose electron-dense material.

8

Myocardial innervation

Basic plan of cardiac innervation

The nerve supply to the heart is capable of modifying the frequency and force of cardiac contraction and it also has the capacity to vary the calibre of the coronary vasculature thus influencing the volume of blood flow to the myocardium. Nerves to the heart are derived from the vagal and sympathetic trunks. Of these, vagal innervation arises from nuclei situated in the medulla oblongata and it comprises afferent and efferent components. The efferent fibres originate from cells in the dorsal nuclei of the vagus and relay in intrinsic cardiac ganglia, the postganglionic fibres of which supply the atrial and ventricular musculature, especially the atrioventricular and sinu-atrial nodes. It was previously supposed that the cardiac ganglia comprise a simple relay system with a presynaptic input of exclusively cholinergic parasympathetic elements and a cholinergic postganglionic output. However, evidence has steadily accumulated to show that the wiring of ganglion cells is more complex and that transmitters other than acetylcholine may be involved as co-transmitters (Hassall & Burnstock, 1986; Burnstock, 1986). Scattered among the neurons of the cardiac ganglia are smaller cells characterised by the presence of monoamine-containing granules in the cytoplasm and these cells are termed small granule-containing cells or, because they manifest characteristic fluorescence on treatment with formaldehyde, small intensely fluorescent cells (SIF cells). Afferent vagal fibres from the heart have their cell bodies mainly in the nodose ganglion and the central processes relay within the medulla oblongata mainly in the nucleus solitarius and dorsal nuclei.

The sympathetic cardiac innervation arises from the intermedio-lateral nucleus in the upper four or five thoracic segments of the spinal cord. The fibres relay in the cervical and upper thoracic ganglia of the sympathetic chain, principally in the stellate ganglion, and postganglionic fibres are distributed to the atrial and ventricular musculature and to the coronary arteries. The pre-ganglionic sympathetic fibres are cholinergic while the postganglio-nic fibres are noradrenergic. The vast majority of these postganglio-nic fibres pass without relay through the intrinsic cardiac ganglia but a small proportion do synapse here on neurons or on SIF cells (Norberg & Sjoqvist, 1966; Burnstock, 1969). Sympathetic nerves also convey sensory fibres from the heart and the relevant cell bodies are believed to lie in the dorsal root ganglia of cervical and thoracic spinal nerves. It is probable that intrinsic cardiac ganglia, like visceral ganglia elsewhere, receive collaterals from sensory nerve fibres which are passing through.

In this chapter, the ultrastructure and organisation of intrinsic cardiac ganglia including SIF cells and non-neuronal supporting components will be discussed followed by a description of terminal nerve ramifications in the myocardium.

Cardiac ganglia

Cardiac ganglia comprise small clumps of neurons, interspersed with SIF cells and supporting cells, which are mainly intramural though some may extend for a short distance along the great vessels. Most of them are apposed to the atria, near the venous openings and within the interatrial septum, while others lie at the base of the aorta near the origins of the coronary arteries. Ganglia related to the ventricles are comparatively rare but Perman (1924) described ventricular ganglia in Cetacea and Artiodactyla and they have also been described from time to time by other authors including Mitchell, Brown & Cookson (1953) in rabbits and primates, Hirsch, Kaiser & Cooper (1965, 1970) in the dog, Anderson & Smith (1971) in cats and Smith (1971) in the human neonate.

There are relatively few papers on the ultrastructure of intrinsic cardiac ganglia although in recent years more have been forthcoming and these have been supplemented by information provided by histochemical and immunocytochemical methods. The earliest substantial account on ultrastructure was provided by Virágh & Porte (1961a,b) and there have been other helpful contributions by Yamauchi (1973), Malor, Taylor, Chesher & Griffin (1974), Zypen, Hasselhorst, Merz & Fillinger (1974), Papka (1976), Ellison & Hibbs (1976), Tay, Wong & Ling (1984a), Shvalev & Sosunov (1985) and Kobayashi, Hassall & Burnstock (1986a). The neurons vary in size from about 12 to 30 μm in diameter and in smaller mammals, such as rodents, they are round or ovoid with a rather smooth outline whereas in larger species, including the cat and monkey, most of them are multipolar. The majority of cells contain a single nucleus of the open vesicular type while a small proportion are binucleate. Most of the chromatin is evenly dispersed and a prominent nucleolus is usually present, often apposed to the nuclear membrane. The cytoplasm contains several dictyosomes of the Golgi apparatus, mitochondria, primary lysosomes and stacks of rough endoplasmic reticulum (Fig. 8.1) can be identified. Amongst these organelles, a few lipofuscin bodies can be seen especially in older animals; these bodies comprise large irregular profiles containing electron-dense patches interspersed with lucent blebs. Numerous neurofilaments are present in the cytoplasm and multivesicular bodies may be found in the periphery of the cell soma especially near points of synaptic contact. In rats and guinea-pigs, the dendrites tend to be short whereas in cats and monkeys they are long and slender (Ellison & Hibbs, 1976). The perikarya and dendrites are surrounded by satellite cell processes (see below).

Histochemical studies confirm that cardiac neurons contain high concentrations of acetylcholinesterase (AChE) in the cytoplasm (Navaratnam, 1965a; Jacobowitz, Cooper & Barner, 1967; Navaratnam, Lewis & Shute, 1968; Ábrahám, 1969; Taylor & Smith, 1971); enzyme staining occurs in the cisterns of the rough endoplasmic reticulum and in the nuclear envelope. The plasma

Fig. 8.1. Perikaryon of neuron located on the posterior wall of the left atrium of an adult rat. The field shows part of the nucleus and numerous cytoplasmic organelles including Golgi apparatus (G), stacks of rough endoplasmic reticulum (ER), mitochondria (M) and secondary lysosomes (L₂). The perikaryon is ensheathed by satellite cell processes (S).

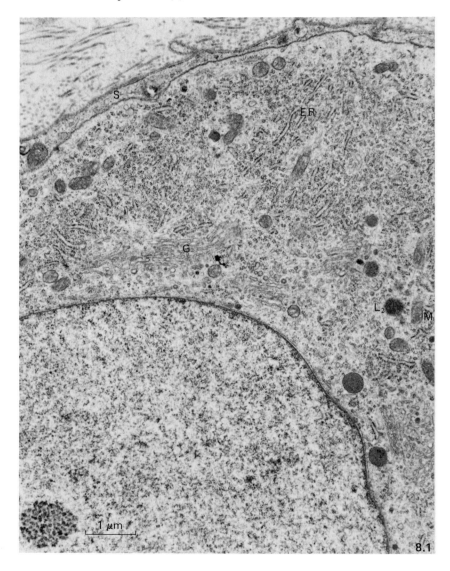

membrane of the perikaryon is generally unstained except where it lies in contact with cholinergic presynaptic terminals. These histochemical observations thus support the view that the majority of cardiac neurons are both cholinergic and cholinoceptive. It is possible, however, that not all neurons fall into this category; Crowe & Burnstock (1982) suggested that some cardiac neurons are purinergic (i.e. use ATP or a similar nucleotide as transmitter) and recent immunocytochemical studies have demonstrated sub-populations of cardiac neurons which are reactive for neuropeptide Y (NPY) or vasoactive intestinal peptide (VIP) (Gu *et al.*, 1984; Weihe, Reinecke & Forssmann, 1984).

Little is known of the functional mechanisms of intracardiac neurons because they are not readily accessible for suitable studies. Some investigations have been conducted on lower vertebrates such as the mud puppy (McMahan & Purves, 1976; Roper, 1976) and there has been a recent limited study by Konishi, Okamoto & Otsuka (1984) of synaptic transmission in a dissected ganglion in the guinea-pig heart. Hassall & Burnstock (1984, 1986) have attempted to circumvent the problem by employing cultured preparations of newborn guinea-pig cardiac ganglia where the majority of cells retain ultrastructural features consistent with that of neurons *in situ* (Kobayashi, Hassall & Burnstock, 1986a). Neurochemical studies on such preparations have confirmed that the neurons are AChE-positive and that subpopulations are immunoreactive for VIP and NPY; however, in addition, a substantial minority of cells in culture have the capacity to take up 5-hydroxytryptamine (5HT) and to synthesise this amine from 5-hydroxytryptophan although such uptake or synthesis has not been demonstrated in neurons *in situ*. Electrophysiological data gathered from cultured neurons suggest that they possess unusually powerful self-regulatory mechanisms and that there are nicotinic as well as muscarinic receptors on these neurons. Autoradiographic studies confirm the presence of large numbers of muscarinic-binding sites on neurons in addition to those on cardiac myocytes. Nevertheless, although such investigations have yielded promising results, more evidence is needed before these findings on cultured preparations can be confidently extrapolated to the normal functions of cardiac neurons. Canale *et al.* (1986) have summarised methods of culturing cardiac muscle and they provide useful information on several features including nerve–muscle interaction.

Presynaptic input to cardiac ganglia

Preganglionic nerves insinuate themselves among the satellite cells and make synaptic contact, mainly *en passant*, with the perikarya and dendrites of cardiac neurons. Ellison & Hibbs (1976) reported that the proportion of axosomatic and axodendritic synapses was determined by the degree of differentiation of dendrites in various species. In species with short dendrites such as the rat and guinea-pig the synapses are predominantly axosomatic whereas in species such as the cat and primates, where the dendrites are long and bear numerous spines, the predominant type is axodendritic.

The majority of synapses are cholinergic (Figs. 8.2, 8.3) and these are usually identified by their content of small round clear vesicles (30–60 nm in diameter) which form the vast majority of the vesicle population even after labelling with 5-hydroxydopamine. Interspersed among the clear vesicles are several mitochondria and a few large granular vesicles (120–250 nm in diameter). The axolemma of these synaptic profiles is AChE-positive. By analogy with other cholinergic neurons it seems certain that the clear vesicles contain acetylcholine while the role of the large granular vesicles is uncertain. Most of the cholinergic terminals degenerate within a few days after bilateral vagotomy but the persistence of a small proportion indicates that some are collaterals from postganglionic axons. Recent studies (Tay, Wong & Ling, 1984*a*) indicate that

Fig. 8.2. Rat left atrial wall showing an axo-somatic synapse. The nerve terminal (A) contains mainly round, clear vesicles and is presumably cholinergic. P, perikaryon of neuron.

Fig. 8.3. Axo-dendritic synapse (presumably cholinergic) on posterior wall of rat left atrium. A, axon terminal; D, dendrite.

Fig. 8.4. Cell containing large granular vesicles (SIF cell) on the back of the left atrium of a rat. Note close apposition to another cell process containing similar granules.

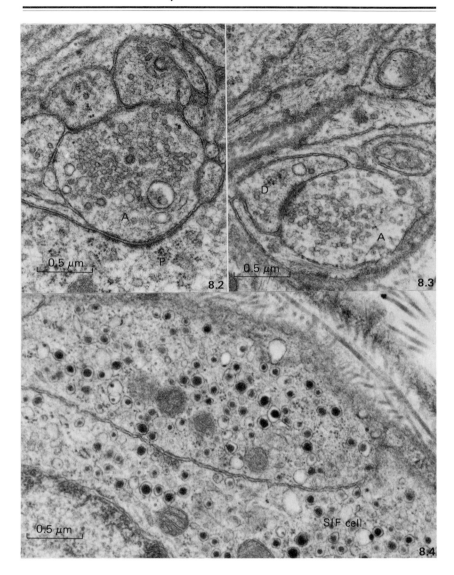

0.5 μm

A

P

8.2

D

A

0.5 μm

8.3

SIF cell

0.5 μm

8.4

transneuronal degenerative changes occur after vagotomy in the macaque monkey but these changes take over a week to set in and do not contribute to the early loss of synapses.

In addition to cholinergic synapses, there is good evidence for the presence of other types of terminals on cardiac neurons. Formaldehyde-induced fluorescence studies under the light microscope (Jacobowitz, 1967; Nielsen & Owman, 1968) have demonstrated the presence of catecholaminergic endings within cardiac ganglia. The likely sources of such endings include (i) post-ganglionic sympathetic fibres coursing through the ganglia and (ii) processes of SIF cells. Ultrastructural studies (Ellison & Hibbs, 1976) have confirmed the presence of noradrenergic varicosities within cardiac ganglia. These varicosities contain small granular vesicles (30–60 nm in diameter) which form the majority of vesicles after labelling with 5-hydroxydopamine, interspersed with a few large granular vesicles and several mitochondria. Even after labelling a small number of vesicles remain clear indicating either that the labelling is incomplete or that they do not contain catecholamine. Degenerative changes can be induced in the granular vesicle-containing terminals as in noradrenergic terminals elsewhere by the administration of 6-hydroxydopamine. Most investigators are inclined to the view that the granular vesicle-containing terminals in cardiac ganglia are derived from sympathetic post-ganglionic nerves and there is little firm proof for input from SIF cells although the latter elements do lie close to the principal neurons.

Other varieties of presynaptic terminals have also been described in cardiac ganglia. These include profiles containing numerous mitochondria and a few large vesicles (200 nm in diameter) with opaque contents but no small vesicles of the granular or agranular type. They resemble terminals described by Burnstock and his colleagues in other tissues such as the gut (Burnstock, 1972) and it has been suggested that they contain ATP or a related purine nucleotide which acts as transmitter. Ellison & Hibbs (1976) have described presynaptic terminals containing flattened clear vesicles interspersed with mitochondria, large granular vesicles and glycogen particles. The functional significance of these terminals is not clear but they resemble inhibitory terminals in the CNS and it is possible that they represent collaterals of afferent fibres coursing through the ganglia.

Although most preganglionic terminals are separated from each other by sheath cell processes, Ellison & Hibbs (1976) have described axo-axonal contacts which often involve apposition of cholinergic and adrenergic terminals. Such preganglionic axo-axonal contacts probably add to the complexities of interaction between adrenergic and cholinergic neurotransmission (Ehinger, Falck & Sporrong, 1970; Levy, 1971); such interaction can occur at both preganglionic and postganglionic levels.

Small granule-containing cells (SIF cells)

The ultrastructure of SIF cells has been described in several mammalian species including rats (Virágh & Porte, 1961a,b; Zypen, 1974; Yamauchi, Yokota & Fujimaki, 1975), guinea-pigs (Ellison & Hibbs, 1974), rabbits (Papka, 1974, 1976), monkeys (Tay, Wong & Ling, 1983) and human foetuses (Dail & Palmer, 1973) as well as in lower vertebrates (see Tay, Wong & Ling, 1983). They occur singly or in small groups of 2–5 cells within cardiac ganglia or very close to them. The cells are small (5–12 μm in diameter) compared to the principal neurons (12–30 μm) and the nucleus is more condensed with more clumped chromatin than in neurons.

The cytoplasm of these cells contains mitochondria, cisterns of rough endoplasmic reticulum, free ribosomes, several Golgi dictyosomes and randomly distributed granular vesicles measuring about 100–125 nm in diameter (Fig. 8.4). The granular nature of these vesicles is not always easy to perceive in unlabelled material but, following the administration of 5-hydroxydopamine, there is marked increase in their prominence. They are distributed throughout the cytoplasm but are more concentrated near the flanks of Golgi complexes and also in the sub-sarcolemmal region. In labelled material, the vesicles contain a large core of electron-dense material which almost fills the cavity but, in some instances, a narrow lucent halo can be discerned between the core and the boundary membrane. Fusion of the vesicular membrane with the plasmalemma is occasionally seen indicating that release of the granular content is effected by exocytosis.

Cell processes containing granular vesicles project for varying distances and some of these processes are carried with axons in the same sheath cells. Perikarya of the SIF cells and their processes often lie close to capillaries indicating that granule contents may be conveyed through the capillary endothelium into the circulation. Such a secretory function for SIF cells has been proposed by Ellison & Hibbs (1974), Papka (1974) and Zypen, Hasselhorst, Merz & Fillinger (1974) but the ultimate function of such a secretion, if it does occur, remains unclear. Braunwald, Harrison & Chidsey (1964) and Papka (1974) suggested that the function could involve acting on the ganglion itself or on nearby cardiac musculature, such as pacemaker cells, or on other more distant tissues.

As pointed out earlier, some SIF cell processes come to lie very near the perikarya and dendrites of the principal neurons (Fig. 8.4), an appearance which led Jacobowitz (1967) to suggest that their activity could affect neuronal firing by a synaptic mechanism. However, most authors have failed to find synaptic contact between SIF cell processes and neurons leaving the existence of such a feedback loop unconfirmed.

Two types of synapses have been observed on SIF cells. These include typical cholinergic terminals with an AChE-positive axolemma and containing clear round vesicles. Jacobowitz (1967) suggested that most of these terminals are derived from post-ganglionic axons but there is evidence, from degenerative changes after cervical vagotomy, that a high proportion are preganglionic parasympathetic axons. The second type of synapse on SIF cells comprises typical noradrenergic terminals containing small dense-core vesicles which can be rendered more conspicuous by labelling with 5-hydroxydopamine.

Non-neuronal supporting elements

Supporting cells in cardiac ganglia include (1) satellite cells related to neuronal perikarya and dendrites, (2) Schwann cells and (3) fibrocytes and mononuclear histiocytes.

Satellite cells are small flattened cells whose cell bodies do not exceed 8 µm in their long diameter. They contain an oval nucleus with fairly dense nucleoplasm and a few clumps of highly condensed chromatin. Processes of these cells form a thin investment layer related to neuronal somata and large dendrites. The internal surface is very closely apposed to the neuronal membrane; the intervening space is narrowed to about 20 nm and excludes the basement lamina which is, however, clearly seen on the external surface of satellite cells. The cytoplasm of satellite cells contains mitochondria, rough endoplasmic reticulum, microfilaments, microtubules and a few small dense bodies (Tay, Wong & Ling, 1984b). Kobayashi, Hassall & Burnstock (1986b) have studied cardiac ganglia of newborn guinea-pigs in culture and have been able to distinguish three types of satellite cell on the basis of their filament content but this variation, which could be due to conditions of culture, has not been confirmed in ganglia *in situ*.

Schwann cells are rather similar to satellite cells though they are more compact in outline and contain less filamentous material. They are readily identifiable by their characteristic relationship to axons, i.e. they contain either several unmyelinated axons or a single myelinated axon. The nuclei are small and contain patches of condensed chromatin within the nucleoplasm. The cytoplasm contains mitochondria, rough endoplasmic reticulum, microtubules and a few microfilaments.

Observations of cardiac ganglia after vagotomy show that Schwann cells and, to a lesser extent, satellite cells can assume scavenger functions (Tay, Wong & Ling, 1984b) necessitated by disintegration of myelin and other material. Mononuclear histiocytes are relatively uncommon in normal material but they increase in number after vagotomy by aggregating near capillaries and undoubtedly contribute to the increased scavenger activity.

Typical fibrocytes are mainly restricted to the capsule surrounding cardiac ganglia but the presence of collagen throughout the ganglion, apart from the narrowed space where satellite cells are apposed to neurons and Schwann cells are apposed to axons, indicates that their activity is more widespread.

Terminal ramifications of nerves

Terminal ramifications of nerves are found (a) in the myocardium, especially in relation to the sinu-atrial and atrioventricular nodes, and (b) in the outer coats of coronary arteries and arterioles down to the precapillary level.

Myocardial nerve terminals

Three main types of axon varicosities can be distinguished in the myocardium.

(i) Typical cholinergic varicosities are found in the atrial myocardium, including the nodes, and to a lesser extent in the ventricular myocardium. These terminals enclose small (30–60 nm in diameter) clear vesicles containing acetylcholine, as well as a few large granular vesicles and numerous mitochondria (Figs. 8.5, 8.6). The axonal membrane stains positively for AChE and the axoplasm contains choline acetyltransferase which can be demonstrated by immunocytochemical techniques. There are no recognisable thickenings on the axolemma or on the sarcolemma of nearby cardiac myocytes; hence it is not easy to recognise with certainty which

Fig. 8.5. A likely cholinergic varicosity in the atrioventricular bundle of an adult hamster. Note the preponderance of clear, round vesicles and a single granular vesicle in the nerve profile.

Fig. 8.6. A likely noradrenergic varicosity in the sinu-atrial node region of an adult rat. A substantial minority of synaptic vesicles are granulated despite lack of labelling with a false transmitter.

Fig. 8.7. Rat sinu-atrial node region showing cholinergic (c) and noradrenergic (na) varicosities. Material labelled with 5-hydroxydopamine which enhances the proportion of granular vesicles in noradrenergic terminals. Picture courtesy of Dr A.S. Ayettey.

Fig. 8.8. A non-cholinergic, non-adrenergic nerve terminal in the sinu-atrial node region of a rat. The predominant organelles in the varicosity are mitochondria, neurotubules, glycogen granules and dense bodies similar in size to the mitochondria.

Fig. 8.9. A non-cholinergic, non-adrenergic nerve profile in the hamster right atrial wall. Mitochondria and dense bodies of similar size are the principal organelles.

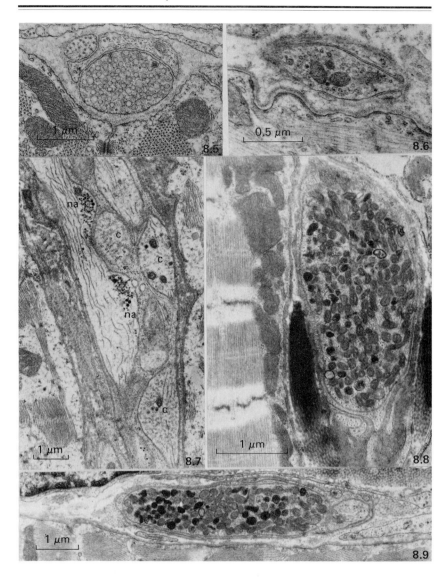

myocytes constitute the effector cells for any particular varicosity, an exercise which is rendered more difficult because the gap between the terminal and the nearest myocyte is highly variable, ranging between 20 and 100 nm. The closest appositions are found in the sinu-atrial and atrioventricular nodes. Autoradiographic techniques have been successfully applied for the localisation of muscarinic receptors in other organs and such receptors have been demonstrated on cardiac myocytes in culture (Lane, Sastre, Law & Salpeter, 1977; Nathanson, 1983). It is likely that in the future such techniques will be able to elucidate how cholinergic terminals are spatially related to muscarinic receptors on cardiac myocytes *in situ*.

(ii) Noradrenergic terminals are found in both atrial and ventricular myocardium and, like cholinergic terminals, they are most frequent in the nodal musculature. These terminals enclose small granular vesicles (30–60 nm) containing noradrenalin, as well as large granular vesicles and mitochondria. The granularity of the small vesicles may not be obvious in unlabelled material (Fig. 8.6) but it becomes conspicuous in a high proportion of the vesicles after an uptake of a false transmitter such as 5-hydroxydopamine (Fig. 8.7). Like cholinergic terminals, there are no presynaptic or post-synaptic membrane thickenings and the gap between terminal and nearest myocyte may be as much as 100 nm; thus, the relationship between nerve terminal and effector myocytes is not clear in most instances. The pharmacological properties of heart muscle indicate that the relevant receptors are of the β_1-adrenergic type.

(iii) Non-cholinergic, non-adrenergic nerves. Varicosities not possessing features of either cholinergic or noradrenergic terminals are not uncommonly found in atrial and ventricular muscle. These varicosities are characterised by their content of densely packed mitochondria (Figs. 8.8, 8.9); there are no small vesicles of the clear or granular variety though some examples contain a few large (200 nm in diameter) vesicles with uniformly opaque material but no granular core and others contain dense lamellar bodies resembling secondary lysosomes. Burnstock (1969) described such varicosities in a variety of organs and proposed that they represent purinergic nerves in which the transmitter is a purine nucleotide, probably ATP. These nerves can be demonstrated by a fluorescent histochemical method using quinacrine (Olson, Ålund & Norberg, 1976). Subsequent ultrastructural studies by Cook & Burnstock (1976) indicated that there is more than one form of non-cholinergic, non-adrenergic terminal and in the myenteric plexus of the guinea-pig they described as many as nine varieties. Immuno-cytochemical and autoradiographic studies show that visceral nerve terminals contain a variety of substances capable of acting as transmitters. These include 5-hydroxytryptamine and γ-aminobutyric acid as well as biologically active peptides such as VIP and NPY. In view of the known presence of VIP and NPY in some cardiac ganglion cells, they probably reside also in a proportion of myocardial nerve terminals (see Burnstock, 1986).

On the other hand, Yamauchi (1973) considered that many of the non-cholinergic, non-adrenergic varicosities in the myocardium are afferent terminals, on the basis that the accumulation of mitochondria without accompanying synaptic vesicles is a feature of sensory terminals in peripheral receptors. Chiba & Yamauchi (1970) estimated that such terminals account for about 5–10% of terminals in human atrial and ventricular myocardium. The axon profiles are large (1.5–3 µm in diameter) and contain glycogen particles as well as dark lamellar bodies in addition to the numerous mitochondria (see Canale et al., 1986). The nerve fibres are enclosed within Schwann cells in common with typical cholinergic and noradrenergic axons. Just over half of the cardiac sensory fibres in the dog have cell bodies in the nodose ganglion of the vagus and probably comprise baroceptor afferents, while the remainder which probably serve pain stimuli have cell bodies in the dorsal root ganglia of cervical and thoracic (mainly T2–T4) spinal nerves.

Cholinergic innervation of ventricular myocardium

Early morphological (see Nonidez, 1939; Cullis & Tribe, 1943) and physiological studies (Drury, 1923; Carlsten, Folkow & Hamberger, 1957; Sarnoff et al., 1960) indicated that ventricular muscle receives no cholinergic innervation. However, evidence has steadily accumulated to show that this view is erroneous. As indicated earlier, several observers have noted the presence of ventricular ganglia in various species. Moreover, histochemical studies have demonstrated the presence of AChE-positive nerves in the ventricular myocardium under the light microscope (Ehinger, Falck, Persson & Sporrong, 1968, in the rabbit, mouse and guinea-pig; Anderson, 1972, in the guinea-pig; Kent, Epstein, Cooper & Jacobowitz, 1974, in man) and electron microscope (Hirano & Ogawa, 1967). Studies of synaptic ultrastructure have confirmed the presence of typical cholinergic varicosities (i.e. containing small clear vesicles resistant to 5-hydroxydopamine labelling) in the ventricular myocardium (Yamauchi, 1973; Ayettey & Navaratnam, 1978b).

The morphological evidence for parasympathetic innervation of ventricular muscle has been corroborated by physiological and pharmacological findings (see Higgins, Vatner & Braunwald, 1973). For example, Eliakim, Bellet, Tawin & Muller (1961), De Geest, Matthew, Zieske & Lipman (1965) and Randall, Priola & Pace (1967) have shown in the dog that vagal stimulation produced a negative inotropic effect in the ventricle as well as in the atrium. Acetylcholine infusion has been shown to cause a similar negative inotropic effect indicating the presence of muscarinic receptors in the ventricle (Levy & Zieske, 1969).

Regional innervation of myocardium

It thus appears that all three types of nerve terminal occur in different regions of the heart but that the density of innervation varies regarding both total innervation and individual types. The density of innervation is highest in the atrioventricular node; for instance in the rat, estimates indicate that there are about 37 nerve varicosities per section of myocyte in the AV-node (Table 8.1), followed by the stem of the AV-bundle (30) and the sinu-atrial node (23). The density of innervation in the general ventricular (12) and atrial myocardium (7) and terminal ramifications of the bundle branches (8) is much lower. That the specialised nodes have a more profuse nerve supply than the general myocardium is not surprising but it is not clear why the atrioventricular node is provided with a higher density than the sinu-atrial node which is the normal pacemaker of the heart.

Estimates of different varieties of nerve terminals in the rat heart indicate that in the atrium, SA-node and AV-node and in the AV-bundle and its ramifications, cholinergic terminals outnumber adrenergic terminals 1.3 : 1 whereas in the ventricular myocardium they are outnumbered 1 : 1.6 by the latter (Table 8.1). Chiba & Yamauchi (1970) indicate a similar preponderance of cholinergic terminals in the atrium and of adrenergic terminals in the ventricle of the human heart.

In general terms, the regional organisation of adrenergic and cholinergic postganglionic terminals in the myocardium can be related to the regulation of cardiac activity. The cardiac rate is normally regulated by the effects of adrenergic and cholinergic nerves on the SA-node, the pacemaker region. Stimulation of cardiac sympathetic nerves, or infusion of adrenalin or noradrenalin, produces a positive chronotropic effect whereas stimulation of the vagus, or infusion of acetylcholine, results in a negative chronotropic effect. However, even the simplest stimula-

Table 8.1 *Distribution of nerve varicosities in rat myocardium after labelling with 5-hydroxydopamine*

Region	Number of varicosities per section of myocyte	Total number of unlabelled varicosities (? cholinergic)	Total number of labelled varicosities (? noradrenergic)	Ratio of unlabelled to labelled varicosities
SA-node	23	1143	869	1.3
Atrial myocardium	7	391	293	1.3
AV-node	37	1568	1116	1.4
AV-bundle	30	1271	1145	1.1
Terminal ramifications of bundle	8	412	306	1.4
Ventricular myocardium	12	413	657	0.6

tion experiments show that the interrelationship between sympathetic and parasympathetic components is more intricate. For example, cessation of adrenergic nerve stimulation is followed by a negative chronotropic effect (Leader, 1963) whilst cessation of cholinergic nerve stimulation is followed by a positive chronotropic effect. A possible explanation of the paradoxical sympathetic effect is that noradrenalin or some other co-transmitter released by sympathetic nerve stimulation acts on closely related cholinergic nerve terminals which exert the delayed negative chronotropic effect. The paradoxical parasympathetic effect could be explained on a similar basis.

While enclosed in the same Schwann cell, axon varicosities are frequently found to be closely apposed; the gap between may be as narrow as 15–20 nm and excludes any process of the Schwann cell, and sometimes even basement membrane is not present. Such appositions have been noted between cholinergic and adrenergic terminals (Ehinger, Falch & Sporrong, 1970) and also between two cholinergic terminals but not between two adrenergic terminals. Ehinger *et al.* have described membrane thickenings at such synaptic appositions but this has not been widely confirmed by other investigators.

Burn & Rand (1959, 1965) suggested that the morphological basis for sympathetic/parasympathetic interactions resides in the presence of cholinergic vesicles within adrenergic terminals. However, this view is no longer tenable because acetylcholine is absent from adrenergic nerves and the basis for peripheral interaction is more likely to lie in the close axo-axonal apposition of cholinergic and adrenergic nerves (see Higgins, Vatner & Braunwald, 1973; Westfall, 1977) at the preganglionic or postganglionic level. The mechanism whereby adrenergic and cholinergic nerves modulate each other is probably useful in protecting the heart against overstimulation of either component. However, the fact that parasympathetic overstimulation can lead to cardiac arrest (Vassalle, 1976; Noble, 1975) shows that such modulatory mechanisms have limitations.

The contractile strength of the heart also is substantially

regulated by autonomic nerves. Adrenergic nerve stimulation causes a positive inotropic effect on both atria and ventricles. However, the negative inotropic effect of the vagus on ventricular myocardium is significantly less than that on atrial myocardium (Harmon & Reeves, 1968; Priola & Fulton, 1969) and pharmacological evidence after acetylcholine infusion supports this view (La Raia & Sonnenblick, 1971). This is partially explained by the presence of fewer cholinergic terminals than adrenergic terminals in the ventricular muscle but it is also likely that ventricular muscle cells are less sensitive to acetylcholine than their atrial counterparts.

Innervation of coronary arteries

There is physiological evidence of the fine control of coronary arteries by adrenergic vasoconstrictor and cholinergic vasodilator nerves (Braunwald, 1966). The direct effects of the vessels are complicated by secondary effects caused by alterations in myocardial activity. For instance, stimulation of sympathetic nerves causes an initial vascular constriction, acting by way of α-adrenergic and β_2-adrenergic receptors, followed by dilatation resulting from enhanced myocardial activity. On the other hand, vagal stimulation causes an increase in blood flow dependent on direct vasodilator effects.

AChE-positive nerve fibres have been demonstrated in the outer coats of coronary arteries in the rat and rabbit (Navaratnam & Palkama, 1965) and there is histochemical evidence for the existence of dual adrenergic and cholinergic innervation of coronary arteries and arterioles in several mammalian species (Schenk & El Badawi, 1968; Nielsen & Owman, 1968; Bojsen-Møller & Tranum-Jensen, 1972).

In an ultrastructural study, Uchizono (1964) described two types of axon terminals, with ultrastructural features of cholinergic and adrenergic types, in the vessels supplying the sinu-atrial region in the dog and rabbit. The terminals lie in the adventitial coat separated by a space of 300–500 nm from the nearest (i.e. outermost) smooth muscle cells. No axon penetration into the tunica media was observed. Similar observations of a loose relationship between axon terminals and smooth muscle of coronary arterioles have been made in the mouse (Moore & Ruska, 1957), rabbit (Parker, 1958; Lever, Ahmed & Irvine, 1965), and rat (Virágh & Porte, 1961a,b; Novi, 1968). These ultrastructural observations are consistent with the view that neurotransmitters may affect the smooth muscle of arteries and arterioles by diffusion across a wide tissue space.

The loose neuroeffector relationship renders vascular smooth muscle more sensitive to the action of more than a single transmitter and these may include not only noradrenalin and acetylcholine but substances such as 5HT and NPY. These substances, which are present in subpopulations of cardiac neurons, have the capacity to induce vasoconstriction; moreover, high concentrations of NPY have been found in coronary vessel walls (Ito & Chiba, 1984; Franco-Cereceda, Lundberg & Dahlof, 1985; Allen et al., 1986).

Occasionally nerve terminals have been found near capillaries in the myocardium as in several other tissues. Forbes, Rennels & Nelson (1977) have suggested that this relationship constitutes innervation of capillaries which can be affected by neurotransmitters diffusing from the terminals. However, the evidence for this view is not strong and it is more likely that the proximity of capillaries to nerve terminals represents the blood supply of the latter rather than innervation of the former.

———

Cardiac ganglia are mainly confined to the atrial wall and to the stems of the main coronary arteries but a few may lie in relation to the ventricles, especially in certain species. They contain neurons, small intensely fluorescent (SIF) cells and supporting cells which include satellite cells, Schwann cells, fibrocytes and histiocytes. The majority of neurons are cholinergic and stain for acetylcholinesterase but there is evidence that some neurons contain peptides such as neuropeptide Y (NPY) and vasoactive intestinal peptide (VIP), purines and 5-hydroxytryptamine. The majority of synapses on ganglion cells are from cholinergic preganglionic parasympathetic fibres but there also are monoaminergic endings derived either from noradrenergic postganglionic sympathetic fibres passing through the ganglia or from SIF cell processes. Axo-axonal contacts, including some between cholinergic and noradrenergic varicosities, occur at preganglionic and postganglionic levels.

SIF cells are smaller than neurons and they contain prominent granular vesicles which are well displayed in material labelled with 5-hydroxydopamine. Their perikarya and processes often lie near capillaries suggesting an endocrine function, but some lie very close to neurons. SIF cells receive endings from preganglionic and postganglionic parasympathetic fibres as well as from noradrenergic sympathetic fibres.

Axon varicosities in the myocardium mainly comprise cholinergic and noradrenergic varieties. Cholinergic axons are preponderant in the atrial wall while noradrenergic terminals are the majority in ventricular muscle. However, there also are terminals which do not resemble either category; some of these are thought to be peptidergic or purinergic while others may be afferent terminals. Nerve varicosities in the coronary arterial walls are widely separated from smooth muscle cells in the tunica media. They are mainly cholinergic or noradrenergic but there is evidence that 5-hydroxytryptamine and NPY also have vasomotor effects on these vessels.

REFERENCES

Ábrahám, A. (1969). *Microscopic Innervation of the Heart and Blood Vessels in Vertebrates including Man.* Oxford: Pergamon.

Abu-Erreisch, G.M. & Sanadi, D.R. (1978). Age related changes in cytochrome concentration of myocardial mitochondria. *Mechanisms of Ageing and Development*, 7, 425–32.

Agakawa, H., Tajiri, T., Hoshino, Y., Kumato, M., Ishino, T., Kosuga, K., Ohishi, K., Hitoshi, T., Tsuda, H. & Koga, M. (1983). Questionable role of glucose-insulin in cardioplegic solution. *Journal of Cardiovascular Surgery*, 24, 215–21.

Akester, A.R. (1981). Intercalated discs, sarcoplasmic reticulum and transitional cells in the heart of the adult domestic fowl (*Gallus gallus domesticus*). *Journal of Anatomy*, 133, 161–79.

Albertini, D.F. & Anderson, E. (1974). The appearance and structure of intercellular connections during the ontogeny of the rabbit ovarian follicle with particular reference to gap junctions. *Journal of Cell Biology*, 63, 234–50.

Albertini, D.F., Fawcett, D.W. & Olds, P.J. (1975). Morphological variations in gap junctions of ovarian granulosa cells. *Tissue and Cell*, 7, 389–402.

Allen, J.M., Gjörstrup, P., Björkman, J-A., Ek, L., Abrahamsson, T. & Bloom, S.R. (1986). Studies on cardiac distribution and function of neuropeptide Y. *Acta physiologica Scandinavica*, 126, 406–11.

Anderson, J.V., Donckier, J., McKenna, W.J. & Bloom, S.R. (1986). The plasma release of atrial natriuretic peptide in man. *Clinical Science*, 71, 151–5.

Anderson, R.H. (1972). The disposition, morphology and innervation of cardiac specialised tissue in the guinea pig. *Journal of Anatomy*, 111, 453–67.

Anderson, R.H. & Smith, R.B. (1971). Feline ventricular ganglion cells. *Nature, New Biology*, 231, 155.

Apstein, C.S., Gravino, F.N. & Haudenschild, C.C. (1983). Determinants of a protective effect of glucose and insulin on the ischemic myocardium. *Circulation Research*, 52, 515–26.

Argüello, C., de la Cruz, M.V. & Gómez, C.S. (1975). Experimental study of the heart tube in the chick embryo. *Journal of Embryology and Experimental Morphology*, 33, 1–11.

Armiger, L.C. & Benson, D.C. (1978). The fine structure of normal canine atrial myocardium, with special reference to mitochondria. *Journal of Molecular and Cellular Cardiology*, 10, 587–92.

Aschoff, L. (1908). Ueber den Glycogengehalt des Reizleitungssystems des Säugetierherzens. (Nach Untersuchungen des Herrn Dr Nagayo). *Verhandlungen der Deutsch pathologischen Gesellschaft*, 12, 150–3.

Ashraf, M. (1978). Ultrastructural alterations in the mitochondrial membranes of ischemic myocardium as revealed by freeze-fracture technique. *Journal of Molecular and Cellular Cardiology*, 10, 535–44.

Ashraf, M., Franklin, D. & Nimmo, L. (1978). Effects of prolonged reperfusion on ischemic myocardium: an ultrastructural evaluation. *Journal of Molecular and Cellular Cardiology*, 10, Suppl. 1, p. 4.

Ashraf, M., White, F. & Bloor, C.M. (1978). Ultrastructural influences of reperfusing dog myocardium with calcium-free blood after coronary artery occlusion. *American Journal of Pathology*, 90, 423–4.

Ayettey, A.S. & Navaratnam, V. (1978*a*) The T-tubule system in the specialized and general myocardium of the rat. *Journal of Anatomy*, 127, 125–40.

Ayettey, A.S. & Navaratnam, V. (1978*b*) 5-OH dopamine labelling of nerve terminals in specialised and general myocardium of the rat. *Journal of Anatomy*, 127, 650.

Ayettey, A.S. & Navaratnam, V. (1980). The fine structure of myocardial cells in the grey seal. *Journal of Anatomy*, 131, 748.

Ayettey, A.S. & Navaratnam, V. (1981). The ultrastructure of myocardial cells in the golden hamster *Cricetus auratus*. *Journal of Anatomy*, 132, 519–24.

Balderman, S.C., Binette, J.P., Chan, A.W.K. & Gage, A.A. (1983). The optimal temperature for preservation of the myocardium during global ischemia. *Annals of Thoracic Surgery*, 35, 605–14.

Balfour, W.E. (1985). On the right lines at last? *Nature*, 314, 226–7.

Ballermann, B.J. & Brenner, B.M. (1986). Role of atrial peptides in body fluid homeostasis. *Circulation Research*, 58, 619–30.

Barden, H. (1970). Relationship of Golgi thiamine pyrophosphatase and lysosomal acid phosphatase to neuromelanin and lipofuscin in cerebral neurons of the aging rhesus monkey. *Experimental Neurology*, 29, 225–40.

Barka, T. (1964). Electron histochemical localization of acid phosphatase activity in the small intestine of the mouse. *Journal of Histochemistry and Cytochemistry*, 12, 229–38.

Barka, T. & Anderson, P.J. (1962). Histochemical methods for acid phosphatase activity in the small intestine of the mouse. *Journal of Histochemistry and Cytochemistry*, 10, 741–53.

Bastian, J. & Nakajima, S. (1974). Action potential in the transverse tubules and its role in the activation of skeletal muscle. *Journal of General Physiology*, 63, 257–78.

Baylor, S.M. & Oetliker, H. (1975). Birefringence experiments on isolated skeletal muscle fibres suggest a possible signal from the sarcoplasmic reticulum. *Nature*, **253**, 97–101.

Bealer, S.L., Haywood, J.R., Gruber, K.A., Buckalew Jr, V.M., Fink, G.D., Brody, M.J. & Johnson, A.K. (1983). Preoptic-hypothalamic periventricular lesions reduce natriuresis to volume expansion. *American Journal of Physiology*, **244**, R51–R57.

Bengele, H.H. (1971). Renal response to blood volume expansion in conscious rats with acute, high spinal cord transection. *Proceedings of the Society of Experimental Biology and Medicine*, **138**, 696–701.

Bennett, M.V.L. & Spray, D.C. (1985). *Gap Junctions* (ed. M.V.L. Bennett & D.C. Spray), pp. 1–3. Cold Spring Harbor Laboratory.

Bezanilla, F. & Horowicz, P. (1975). Fluorescence intensity changes associated with contractile activation in frog sartorius muscle stained with Nile Blue A. *Journal of Physiology*, **246**, 709–35.

Blaineau-Peyretti, S. & Nicaise, G. (1976). Strontium accumulation in atrial muscle cells. *Journal de Microscopie et de Biologie cellulaire*, **26**, 127–32.

Blayney, L. (1983). Calcium sarcoplasmic reticulum. In *Cardiac Metabolism* (ed. A.J. Drake-Holland & M.I.M. Noble), pp. 19–47. Chichester: John Wiley & Sons.

Blennerhassett, M.G. & Caveney, S. (1983). How selective is gap junctional permeability at the compartment border? *Journal of Cell Biology*, **97**, 125a.

Boink, A.B.T.J., Ruigrok, T.J.C., Maas, A.H.J. & Zimmerman, A.N.E. (1978). Myocardial recovery after calcium-free perfusion of isolated rat hearts at different temperatures. *Journal of Molecular and Cellular Cardiology*, **10**, Suppl. 1, p. 12.

Bojsen-Møller, F. & Tranum-Jensen, J. (1972). Rabbit heart nodal tissue, sinuatrial ring bundle and atrioventricular connections identified as a neuromuscular system. *Journal of Anatomy*, **112**, 367–82.

Bompiani, G.D., Roniller, C. & Hatt, P.Y. (1959). Le tisu de conduction de coeur chez le rat. Étude au microscope électronique. *Archives des Maladies du Coeur et des Vaisseaux*, **52**, 1257–74.

Braunwald, E. (1966). Heart. *Annual Review of Physiology*, **28**, 227–66.

Braunwald, E., Harrison, D.C. & Chidsey, C.A. (1964). The heart as an endocrine organ. *American Journal of Medicine*, **36**, 1–4.

Bruce, T.A. & Myers, J.T. (1973). Myocardial lipid metabolism in ischemia and infarction. *Recent Advances in Studies on Cardiac Structure and Metabolism*, vol. 3 (ed. N.S. Dhalla), pp. 773–80. Baltimore: University Park Press.

Burn, J.H. & Rand, M. (1959). Sympathetic postganglionic mechanism. *Nature*, **184**, 163.

Burn, J.H. & Rand, M.J. (1965). Acetylcholine in adrenergic transmission. *Annual Review of Pharmacology*, **5**, 163–82.

Burnstock, G. (1969). Evolution of autonomic innervation of visceral and cardiovascular systems in vertebrates. *Pharmacological Reviews*, **21**, 247–324.

Burnstock, G. (1972). Purinergic nerves. *Pharmacological Reviews*, 24, 509–81.

Burnstock, G. (1986). Autonomic neuromuscular junctions: current developments and future directions. *Journal of Anatomy*, 146, 1–30.

Butcher, R.G. (1983). Enzyme histochemistry of the myocardium. In *Cardiac Metabolism* (ed. A.J. Drake-Holland & M.I.M. Noble), pp. 445–69. Chichester: John Wiley & Sons.

Caesar, R., Edwards, G.A. & Ruska, H. (1958). Electron microscopy of the impulse conducting system of the sheep heart. *Zeitschrift für Zellforschung und mikroskopische Anatomie*, 48, 698–719.

Canale, E.D., Campbell, G.R., Smolich, J.J. & Campbell, J.H. (1986). *Cardiac Muscle*. Berlin, Heidelberg: Springer-Verlag.

Cano, J., Hervas, J.P. & Machado, A. (1981). Myelin-like inclusions in maturing and senescent muscle cells of rat myocardium. *Mechanisms of Ageing and Development*, 17, 131–40.

Cantin, M. & Genest, J. (1986). The heart as an endocrine gland. *Scientific American*, 254, 62–7.

Cantin, M. & Huet, M. (1975). Chemical nature of atrial specific granules. In *Recent Advances in Studies on Cardiac Structure and Metabolism. Pathophysiology and Morphology of Myocardial Cell Alterations*, vol. 6 (ed. A. Fleckenstein & G. Rona), pp. 313–22. Baltimore: University Park Press.

Cantin, M., Timm-Kennedy, M., El-Khatib, E., Huet, M. & Yunge, L. (1979). Ultrastructural cytochemistry of atrial muscle cells. VI. Comparative study of specific granules in right and left atrium of various animal species. *Anatomical Record*, 193, 55–69.

Carlsten, A., Folkow, B. & Hamberger, C.A. (1957). Cardiovascular effects of direct vagal stimulation in man. *Acta physiologica Scandinavica*, 41, 68–76.

Carswell, F., Hainsworth, R. & Ledsome, J.R. (1970). The effects of left atrial distension upon urine flow from the isolated perfused kidney. *Journal of Experimental Physiology*, 55, 173–82.

Caspar, D.L.D., Goodenough, D.A., Makowski, L. & Phillips, W.C. (1977). Gap junction structures. I. Correlated electron microscopy and X-ray diffraction. *Journal of Cell Biology*, 74, 605–28.

Cavoto, F.V., Kelleher, G.J. & Roberts, J. (1974). Electrophysiological changes in the rat atrium with age. *Journal of Physiology*, 226, 1293–7.

Challice, C.E. (1965). Studies on the microstructure of the heart. I. The sino-atrial node and sino-atrial ring bundle. *Journal of the Royal Microscopical Society*, 85, 1–21.

Challice, C.E. & Virágh, S. (1973). The embryologic development of the mammalian heart. In *Ultrastructure of the Mammalian Heart* (ed. C.E. Challice & S. Virágh), chapter 3, pp. 91–126. New York: Academic Press.

Chapeau, C., Gutkowska, J., Schiller, P., Milne, R.W., Thibault, G., Garcia, R., Genest, J. & Cantin, M. (1985). Localization of immunoreactive synthetic atrial natriuretic factor (ANF) in the heart of various animal species. *Journal of Histochemistry and Cytochemistry*, 33, 541–50.

Chen, Y-F. & Lin, Y-T. (1984). Comparison of blood cardioplegia to electrolyte cardioplegia on the effectiveness of preservation of right atrial myocardium: mitochondrial morphometric study. *Annals of Thoracic Surgery*, **39**, 134–8.

Cheng, Y.P. (1971). The ultrastructure of the rat sino-atrial node. *Acta anatomica Nippon*, **46**, 339–58.

Chiba, T. (1973). Electron microscopic and histochemical studies on the synaptic vesicles in mouse vas deferens and atrium after 5-hydroxydopamine administration. *Anatomical Record*, **176**, 35–48.

Chiba, T. & Yamauchi, A. (1970). On the fine structure of nerve terminals in the human myocardium. *Zeitschrift für Zellforschung und mikroskopische Anatomie*, **108**, 324–38.

Chio, K.S. & Tappel, A.L. (1969). Inactivation of ribonuclease and other enzymes by peroxidasing lipids and by malonaldehyde. *Biochemistry*, **8**, 2827–32.

Chiodi, V. & Bartolami, R. (1967). *The Conducting System of the Vertebrate Heart*. Bologna: Edizioni Calderini.

Colborn, G.L. & Garsey Jr, E. (1972). Electron microscopy of the sino-atrial node of the squirrel monkey (*Saimiri sciureus*). *Journal of Molecular and Cellular Cardiology*, **4**, 525–36.

Colcolough, H.L., Hack, M.H., Helmy, F.M., Vaugh, G.E. & Veith, D.C. (1972). Some histochemical, biochemical and morphological observations relating to lipofuscin and mitochondria. *Acta Histochemica*, **43**, 98–109.

Coleman, R., Silbermann, M., Gerschon, D. & Reznick, A. (1982). An ultrastructural study of lipofuscin and macrophages in the ventricular myocardium of ageing and endurance-trained mice. *Biology of the Cell*, **46**, 207–10.

Cook, R.D. & Burnstock, G. (1976). The ultrastructure of Auerbach's plexus in the guinea-pig. I. Neuronal elements. *Journal of Neurocytology*, **5**, 171–94.

Crowe, R. & Burnstock, G. (1982). Fluorescent histochemical localisation of quinacrine-positive neurones in the guinea-pig and rabbit atrium. *Cardiovascular Research*, **16**, 384–90.

Cullis, W. & Tribe, E.M. (1943). Distribution of nerves in the heart. *Journal of Physiology*, **46**, 141–50.

Dahl, G. & Isenberg, G. (1980). Decoupling of heart muscle cells, correlation with increased cytoplasmic calcium activity and with changes of nexus ultrastructure. *Journal of Membrane Biology*, **53**, 63–75.

Dail, W.G. Jr. & Palmer, G.E. (1973). Localization and correlation of catecholamine-containing cells with adenyl cyclase and phosphodiesterase activities in the human fetal heart. *Anatomical Record*, **177**, 265–88.

Davis, C.L. (1927). Development of the human heart from its first appearance to the stage found in embryos of twenty paired somites. *Contributions to Embryology*, **19**, 245–84.

De Boer, L.W.V., Rude, R.E., Kloner, R.A., Ingwall, J.S., Maroko, P.R., Davis, M.A. & Braunwald, E. (1983). A flow- and time-dependent index of ischemic injury after experimental coronary occlusion and reperfusion. *Proceedings of the National Academy of Sciences, U.S.A.*, **80**, 5784–8.

De Bold, A.J. (1979). Heart atria granularity effects of changes in water electrolyte balance. *Proceedings of the Society of Experimental Biology and Medicine*, **161**, 508–11.

De Bold, A.J. (1986). Atrial natriuretic factor: an overview. *Federation Proceedings*, **45**, 2081–5.

De Bold, A.J. & Bencosme, S.A. (1973). Studies of the relationship between the catecholamine distribution in the atrium and the specific granules present in atrial muscle cells. II. Studies on the sedimentation pattern of atrial noradrenalin and adrenalin. *Cardiovascular Research*, **7**, 364–9.

De Bold, A.J., Borenstein, H.B., Veress, A.T. & Sonnenberg, H. (1981). A rapid and potent natriuretic response to intravenous injection of atrial myocardial extract in rats. *Life Science*, **28**, 89–94.

De Duve, C. (1964). From cytases to lysosomes. *Federation Proceedings*, **23**, 1045–9.

De Fellice, L.J. & Challice, C.E. (1969). Anatomical and ultrastructural study of the electrophysiological atrioventricular node of the rabbit. *Circulation Research*, **24**, 457–74.

De Geest, H., Matthew, N.L., Zieske, H. & Lipman, R.I. (1965). Depression of ventricular contractility by stimulation of the vagus nerves. *Circulation Research*, **17**, 222–35.

De Haan, R.L. (1964). Cell interactions and orientated movements during development. *Journal of Experimental Zoology*, **157**, 127–38.

De Haan, R.L. (1965). Morphogenesis of the vertebrate heart. In *Organogenesis* (ed. R.L. De Haan & H. Ursprung), pp. 377–419. New York: Academic Press.

De Wardener, H.E. & Clarkson, E.M. (1985). Concept of natriuretic hormone. *Physiological Reviews*, **65**, 659–759.

Decker, R.S. (1974). Lysosomal packaging in differentiating and degenerating anuran lateral motor column neurons. *Journal of Cell Biology*, **61**, 559–612.

Decker, R.S. (1976). Hormonal regulation of gap-junction differentiation. *Journal of Cell Biology*, **69**, 669–85.

Decker, R.S. & Friend, D.S. (1974). Assembly of gap junctions during amphibian neurulation. *Journal of Cell Biology*, **62**, 32–47.

Derietzel, R., Leibstein, A., Frixen, U., Janssen-Timmen, U., Traub, O. & Willecke, K. (1984). Gap junctions in several tissues share antigenic determinants with liver gap junctions. *E.M.B.O. Journal*, **3**, 2261–70.

Dewey, M.M. (1969). The structure and function of the intercalated disc in vertebrate cardiac muscle. *Experientia*, Suppl. 15, 10–28.

Dewey, M.M. & Barr, L. (1964). A study of the structure and distribution of the nexus. *Journal of Cell Biology*, **23**, 553–85.

Dhoot, G.K. & Perry, S.V. (1979). Distribution of polymorphic forms of troponin components and tropomyosin in skeletal muscle. *Nature*, **278**, 714–18.

Dreifuss, J.J., Girardier, L. & Forssmann, W.G. (1966). Étude de la propagation de l'excitation dans la ventricule de rat au moyen de solutions hypertoniques. *Pflügers Archiv*, **292**, 13–33.

Drury, A.N. (1923). The influence of vagal stimulation upon the force of contraction and the refractory period of ventricular muscle in the dog's heart. *Heart*, **10**, 405–15.

Ebashi, S. (1963). Third component participating in the superprecipitation of 'natural actomyosin'. *Nature*, **200**, 1010.

Eberth, C.J. (1866). Die Elemente der quergestreifeten Muskeln. *Archiv für pathologsiche Anatomie und Physiologie*, **37**, 100–24.

Edonte, Y., van der Merwe, E., Sanan, D., Kotzé, J.C.N., Steinmann, C. & Lochner, A. (1983). Normothermic ischemic cardiac arrest of the isolated working rat heart: effects of time and reperfusion on myocardial ultrastructure, mitochondrial oxidative function and mechanical recovery. *Circulation Research*, **53**, 663–78.

Ehinger, B., Falck, B., Persson, H. & Sporrung, B. (1968). Adrenergic and cholinesterase-containing neurons of the heart. *Histochemie*, **16**, 197–205.

Ehinger, B., Falck, B. & Sporrong, B. (1970). Possible axo-axonal synapses between adrenergic and cholinergic nerve terminals. *Zeitschrift für Zellforschung und mikroskopsiche Anatomie*, **107**, 508–21.

Eliakim, M., Bellet, S., Tawin, E. & Muller, O. (1961). Effect of vagal stimulation and acetylcholine on the ventricle. Studies in dogs with complete heart block. *Circulation Research*, **9**, 1372–9.

Elias, P.M. & Friend, D.S. (1976). Vitamin-A-induced mucous metaplasia, an in vitro system for modulating tight and gap junction differentiation. *Journal of Cell Biology*, **68**, 173–88.

Ellison, J.P. & Hibbs, R.C. (1974). Catecholamine-containing cells of the guinea-pig heart: an ultrastructural study. *Journal of Molecular and Cellular Cardiology*, **6**, 17–26.

Ellison, J.P. & Hibbs, R.G. (1976). An ultrastructural study of mammalian cardiac ganglia. *Journal of Molecular and Cellular Cardiology*, **8**, 89–101.

Endo, M. (1977). Calcium release from the sarcoplasmic reticulum. *Physiological Reviews*, **57**, 71–108.

Epstein, M.L. & Gilula, N.B. (1977). A study of communication specificity between cells in culture. *Journal of Cell Biology*, **75**, 769–87.

Essner, E. & Novikoff, A.B. (1960). Human hepatocellular pigments and lysosomes. *Journal of Ultrastructure Research*, **3**, 374–91.

Essner, E. & Novikoff, A.B. (1961). Localization of acid phosphatase activity in hepatic lysosomes by means of electron microscopy. *Journal of Biophysics, Biochemistry and Cytology*, **9**, 773–84.

Essner, E., Novikoff, A.B. & Quintana, N. (1965). Nucleoside phosphatase activities in rat cardiac muscle. *Journal of Cell Biology*, **25**, 201–15.

Fabiato, F. (1977). Calcium release from the sarcoplasmic reticulum. *Circulation Research*, **40**, 119–29.

Fater, D.C., Schultz, H.D., Sundet, W.D., Mapes, J.S. & Goetz, K.L. (1982).

Effects of left atrial stretch in cardiac denervated and intact conscious dogs. *American Journal of Physiology*, **242**, H1056–H1064.

Fawcett, D.W. & McNutt, N.S. (1969). The ultrastructure of the cat myocardium. 1. Ventricular papillary muscle. *Journal of Cell Biology*, **42**, 1–45.

Feldman, M.L. & Navaratnam, V. (1981). Ultrastructural changes in atrial myocardium of the ageing rat. *Journal of Anatomy*, **133**, 7–17.

Ferrans, V.J., Buja, L.M., Levitsky, S., Williams, W.H., McIntosh, C.L. & Roberts, W.C. (1972). Cardiac preservation: a morphologic study. In *Recent Advances in Studies on Cardiac Structure and Metabolism*, vol. 1 (ed. E. Bajusz & G. Rona), pp. 351–75. Baltimore: University Park Press.

Fischer, V.W. & Barner, H.B. (1978). Ultrastructural integrity of human ventricular myocardium following cardioplegic arrest. *Annals of Thoracic Surgery*, **27**, 49–54.

Flameng, W., Suy, R., Schwartz, F., Borgers, M., Piessens, J., Thone, F., Van Ermen, H. & De Geest, H. (1981). Ultrastructural correlates of left ventricular contraction abnormalities in patients with chronic ischemic heart disease; determinants of reversible segmental asynergy postrevascularization surgery. *American Heart Journal*, **102**, 846–57.

Flynn, T.G., De Bold, M.L. & De Bold, A.J. (1983). The amino acid sequence of an atrial peptide with potent natriuretic and diuretic properties. *Biochemical and Biophysical Research Communications*, **117**, 859–65.

Fonda, M.L., Herbener, G.H. & Cuddihee, R.W. (1983). Biochemical and morphometric studies of the heart, liver and skeletal muscle from the hibernating, arousing and aroused big brown bat (*Eptisecus fucus*). *Comparative Biochemistry and Physiology*, **76B**, 355–63.

Forbes, M.S., Hawkey, L.A. & Sperelakis, N. (1984). The transverse-axial tubular system (TATS) of mouse myocardium: its morphology in the developing and adult animal. *American Journal of Anatomy*, **170**, 143–62.

Forbes, M.S., Rennels, M.L. & Nelson, E. (1977). Innervation of myocardial microcirculation. Terminal autonomic axons associated with capillary and postcapillary venules in mouse heart. *American Journal of Anatomy*, **149**, 71–91.

Forbes, M.S. & Sperelakis, N. (1977). Myocardial couplings: their structural variations in the mouse. *Journal of Ultrastructure Research*, **58**, 50–65.

Forssmann, W.G. & Girardier, L. (1970). A study of the T-system in rat heart. *Journal of Cell Biology*, **44**, 1–19.

Franco-Cereceda, A., Lundberg, J.M. & Dahlof, C. (1985). Neuropeptide Y and sympathetic control of heart contractility and coronary vascular tone. *Acta physiologica Scandinavica*, **124**, 361–9.

Frank, A.L. & Christianson, A.K. (1968). Localization of acid phosphatase in lipofuscin granules and possible autophagic vacuoles in interstitial cells of the guinea pig testis. *Journal of Cell Biology*, **36**, 1–13.

Frank, J.S., Rich, T.L., Beydler, S. & Kreman, M. (1982). Calcium depletion in rabbit myocardium. Ultrastructure of the sarcolemma and correlation with the calcium paradox. *Circulation Research*, **51**, 117–30.

Franzini-Armstrong, C. (1974). Freeze-fracture of skeletal muscle from the tarantula spider. Structural differentiations of sarcoplasmic reticulum and transverse tubular system membranes. *Journal of Cell Biology*, **61**, 501–13.

Friend, D.S. & Gilula, N.B. (1972). Variations in tight and gap junctions in mammalian tissues. *Journal of Cell Biology*, **53**, 758–76.

Fundoianu-Dayan, D., Abrahami, I., Buchner, A. & Gorsky, M. (1985). Lipofuscins in human pectoral muscles. *International Workshop of Age Pigments: Biological Markers in Aging and Environmental Stress*, p. 18. Napoli: Castello Giusso.

Ganote, C-E. (1986). Contracture as a mediator of calcium paradox (CP) and CP-like injury. *Journal of Molecular and Cellular Cardiology*, **18**, Suppl. 1, p. 37.

Garcia, R., Cantin, M., Thibault, G., Ong, H. & Genest, J. (1982). Relationship of specific granules to the natriuretic and diuretic activity of rats. *Experientia*, **38**, 1071–3.

Gauer, O.H. & Henry, J.P. (1976). Neurohormonal control of plasma volume. In *Cardiovascular Physiology II* (ed. A.C. Guyton & A.W. Cowley). Baltimore: University Park Press.

Gavin, J.B., Thomson, R.W., Humphrey, S.M. & Herdson, P.B. (1983). Changes in vascular morphology associated with the no-reflow phenomenon in ischemic myocardium. *Virchows Archiv A, Pathological Anatomy and Histology*, **399**, 325–32.

Gedigk, P. & Bontke, E. (1956). Über den Nachweis von hyrolischen Enzymen in Lipopigmentum. *Zeitschrift für Zellforschung und mikroskopische Anatomie*, **44**, 495–518.

Ghosh, A., Bern, H.A., Ghosh, J. & Nishioka, R.S. (1962). Nature of the inclusions in the lumbosacral neurons of birds. *Anatomical Record*, **143**, 195–218.

Giaume, C. & Korn, H. (1985). Junctional voltage-dependence at the crayfish rectifying synapse. In *Gap Junctions* (ed. M.V.L. Bennett & D.C. Spray), pp. 367–79. Cold Spring Harbor Laboratory.

Gilmore, J.P. & Daggett, W.M. (1966). Response of the chronic cardiac denervated dog to acute volume expansion. *American Journal of Physiology*, **210**, 509–12.

Glees, P. (1985). Removal of osmiophilic waste products from neurons. *International Workshop on Age Pigments: Biological Markers in Aging and Environmental Stress*, p. 19. Napoli: Castelo Giusso.

Goldberg, P.B. (1978). Cardiac function of Fischer 344 rats in relation to age. In *Aging in Muscle* (ed. G. Kaldov & W.J. DiBattista), pp. 87–100. New York: Raven Press.

Goldfischer, S. (1982). The internal reticular apparatus of Gamillo Golgi; a complex, heterogeneous organelle, enriched in acid, neutral and alkaline phosphatase and involved in glycosylation, secretion, membrane flow, lysosome formation and intercellular digestion. *Journal of Histochemistry and Cytochemistry*, **30**, 717–33.

Goldfischer, S., Villaverde, H. & Forschirm, R. (1966). The demonstration of acid hydrolase, thermostable reduced diphosphopyridine nucleotide tetrazolium reductase and peroxidase activities in human lipofuscin pigment granules. *Journal of Histochemistry and Cytochemistry*, **14**, 641–52.

Goldstein, M.A. & Murphy, D.L. (1983). A morphometric analysis of ischemic canine myocardium with and without reperfusion. *Journal of Molecular and Cellular Cardiology*, **15**, 325–34.

Goldstein, M.A., Shroeter, J.P. & Sass, R.L. (1977). Optical diffraction of the Z-lattice in canine cardiac muscle. *Journal of Cell Biology*, **75**, 818–36.

Goodenough, D.A. (1975). Methods for the isolation and structural characterization of hepatocyte gap junctions. In *Methods in Membrane Biology*, vol. 3 (ed. E.B. Korn), pp. 51–80. New York: Plenum Press.

Görlach, G., Scheld, H.H., Mulch, J., Schaper, J. & Hehrlein, F.W. (1986). Ultrastructure of the human myocardium after intermittent ischemia compared to cardioplegia. In *Myocardial and Skeletal Muscle Bioenergetics* (ed. N. Brautbar), pp. 439–49. New York: Plenum Press.

Goss, C.M. (1938). The first contractions of the heart in rat embryos. *Anatomical Record*, **70**, 505–24.

Goss, C.M. (1952). Development of the median coordinated ventricle from the lateral hearts in rat embryos with three to six somites. *Anatomical Record*, **112**, 761–96.

Gros, D. & Challice, C.E. (1975). The coating of mouse myocardiac cells. A cytochemical electron microscopical study. *Journal of Histochemistry and Cytochemistry*, **23**, 727–44.

Gros, D., Mocquard, J.P., Challice, C.E. & Schrevel, J. (1978). Formation and growth of gap junctions in mouse myocardium during ontogenesis; a freeze-cleave study. *Journal of Cell Science*, **30**, 45–61.

Gros, D.B., Nicholson, B.J. & Revel, J.P. (1983). Comparative analysis of the gap junction protein from rat heart and liver. *Cell*, **35**, 539–49.

Gu, J., Polak, J.M., Allen, J.M., Huang, W.M., Sheppard, M.N., Tatemoto, K. & Bloom, S.R. (1984). High concentrations of a novel peptide, Neuropeptide Y, in the innervation of the mouse and rat heart. *Journal of Histochemistry and Cytochemistry*, **32**, 467–72.

Harden III, W.R., Barlow, C.H., Soriano, R., Mela, L. & Harken, A.H. (1978). Epicardial NADH fluorescence in the evaluation of myocardial ischemia-ultrastructural and mitochondrial correlation. *Federation Proceedings*, **37**, 899.

Harmon, M.A. & Reeves, T.J. (1968). Effect of efferent vagal stimulation on atrial and ventricular function. *American Journal of Physiology*, **215**, 1210–17.

Harrison, R.J. & Ridgway, S.H. (1976). *Deep Diving in Mammals*. Durham: Meadowfield Press.

Hasan, M. & Glees, P. (1972). Genesis and possible dissolution of neuronal lipofuscin. *Gerontologia*, **18**, 217–36.

Hassall, C.J.S. & Burnstock, G. (1984). Neuropeptide Y-like immunoreactivity in cultured intrinsic neurones of the heart. *Neuroscience Letters*, **52**, 111–15.

Hassall, L.J.S. & Burnstock, G. (1986). Intrinsic neurones and associated cells of the guinea-pig heart in culture. *Brain Research*, **364**, 102–13.

Hayashi, K. (1962). An electron microscope study on the conduction system of the cow heart. *Japanese Circulation Journal*, **26**, 765–842.

Hayashi, S. (1971). Electron microscopy of the heart conducting system of the dog. *Archives of Histology, Japan*, **33**, 67–86.

Hearse, D.J., Braimbridge, M.V. & Jynge, P. (1981). *Protection of the Ischemic Myocardium: Cardioplegia*. New York: Raven Press.

Heller, L.G. & Whitehorn, W.V. (1972). Age associated alterations in myocardial contractile properties. *American Journal of Physiology*, **222**, 1613–19.

Henderson, D., Eibl, H. & Weber, K. (1979). Structure and biochemistry of mouse hepatic gap junctions. *Journal of Molecular Biology*, **132**, 193–218.

Hendley, D.D. & Strehler, B.L. (1965). Enzyme activities of lipofuscin age pigments; comparative histochemical and biochemical studies. *Biochimica et Biophysica Acta*, **99**, 406–17.

Herbener, G.H. (1976). A morphometric study of age-dependent changes in mitochondrial populations in mouse liver and heart. *Journal of Gerontology*, **31**, 8–12.

Herscher, L.L., Siegel, R.J., Said, J.W., Edwalds, G.M., Moran, M.M. & Fishbein, M.C. (1984). Distribution of LDH-1 in normal, ischemic and necrotic myocardium. An immunoperoxidase study. *American Journal of Clinical Pathology*, **31**, 198–203.

Hertsens, R.C., Bernaert, I., Jonian, I. & Jacob, W.A. (1986). Immunocytochemical investigation of native matrix granules of the rat heart mitochondrion. *Journal of Ultrastructure and Molecular Structure Research*, **94**, 1–15.

Hertzberg, E.L., Anderson, B.J., Friedlander, M. & Gilula, N.B. (1982). Comparative analysis of the major polypeptides from liver gap junctions and lens fibre junctions. *Journal of Cell Biology*, **92**, 53–9.

Hertzberg, E.L. & Gilula, N.B. (1979). Isolation and characterization of gap junctions from rat liver. *Journal of Biology and Chemistry*, **254**, 2138–47.

Hertzberg, E.L. & Skibbens, R.V. (1984). A protein homologous to the 27,000 dalton liver gap junction protein is present in a wide variety of species and tissues. *Cell*, **39**, 61–9.

Hertzberg, E.L. & Spray, D.C. (1985). Studies of gap junctions: biochemical analysis and use of antibody probes. In *Gap Junctions* (ed. M.V.L. Bennett & D.C. Spray), pp. 57–65. Cold Spring Harbor Laboratory.

Hibbs, R.G. & Ferrans, V.J. (1969). An ultrastructural and histochemical study of rat atrial myocardium. *American Journal of Anatomy*, **124**, 251–80.

Hicks, L. & Fahimi, H.D. (1977). Peroxisomes (microbodies) in the myocardium of rodents and primates. A comparative ultrastructural cytochemical study. *Cell and Tissue Research*, **175**, 467–82.

Higgins, C.B., Vatner, S.F. & Braunwald, E. (1973). Parasympathetic control of the heart. *Pharmacological Reviews*, **25**, 119–55.

Hirakow, R. & De Haan, R.L. (1970). Synchronization and the formation of nexal junctions between isolated chick embryonic heart myocytes beating in culture. *Journal of Cell Biology*, **47**, 88a.

Hirakow, R., Gotoh, T. & Watanabe, T. (1980). Quantitative studies on the ultrastructural differentiation and growth of mammalian cardiac muscle cells. *Acta Anatomica*, **108**, 144–52.

Hirano, H. & Ogawa, K. (1967). Ultrastructural localization of cholinesterase activity in nerve endings in the guinea pig heart. *Journal of Electronmicroscopy*, **16**, 313–21.

Hirsch, E.F., Kaiser, G.C. & Cooper, T. (1965). Experimental heart block in the dog. III. Distribution of the vagus and sympathetic nerves in the septum. *Archives of Pathology*, **79**, 441–51.

Hirsch, E.F., Kaiser, G.C. & Cooper, T. (1970). The innervation of the canine heart. In *The Innervation of the Vertebrate Heart* (ed. E.F. Hirsch), pp. 80–101. Springfield, Ill.: C.C. Thomas.

Holtzman, E.A., Novikoff, A.B. & Villaverde, H. (1967). Lysosomes and GERL in normal and chromatolytic neurons of the rat ganglion nodosum. *Journal of Cell Biology*, **33**, 419–35.

Huet, M., Benchimol, S., Costonguay, Y. & Cantin, M. (1974). Ultrastructural cytochemistry of atrial muscle cells. III. Reactivity of specific granules in man. *Histochemie*, **41**, 87–106.

Huet, M. & Cantin, M. (1974a). Ultrastructural cytochemistry of atrial muscle cells. I. Characterization of carbohydrate content of specific granules. *Laboratory Investigations*, **30**, 514–24.

Huet, M. & Cantin, M. (1974b). Ultrastructural cytochemistry of atrial muscle cells. II. Characterization of the protein content of specific granules. *Laboratory Investigations*, **30**, 525–32.

Hülsmann, W.C.. & Stam, H. (1979). Lipolysis in heart and adipose tissue: effects of inhibition of glycogenolysis and uncoupling of oxidative phosphorylation. *Biochemical and Biophysical Research Communications*, **88**, 867–72.

Humphrey, S.M., Thomson, R.W. & Gavin, J.B. (1984). The influence of no-reflow on reperfusion and reoxygenation damage and enzyme release from anoxic and ischemic isolated rat hearts. *Journal of Molecular and Cellular Cardiology*, **16**, 915–30.

Humphrey, S.M. & Vanderwee, S.M. (1986). Factors affecting the development of contraction band necrosis during reperfusion of the isolated isovolumic rat heart. *Journal of Molecular and Cellular Cardiology*, **18**, 319–30.

Huxley, H.E. (1973). Molecular basis of contraction in cross-striated muscles. In *The Structure and Function of Muscle*, 2nd edn, vol. 1 (ed. G.H. Bourne), pp. 301–87. New York: Academic Press.

Huxley, A.F. & Taylor, R.E. (1958). Local activation of striated muscle fibres. *Journal of Physiology*, **144**, 426–41.

Ito, T. & Chiba, S. (1984). Responses of isolated canine intermediate auricular arteries to 5-hydroxytryptamine and methysergide. *European Journal of Pharmacology*, **104**, 105–9.

Jacobowitz, D. (1967). Histochemical studies of the relationship of chromaffin cells and adrenergic nerve fibres to the cardiac ganglia of several species. *Journal of Pharmacology and Experimental Therapeutics*, **158**, 227–40.

Jacobowitz, D., Cooper, T. & Barner, H.B. (1967). Histochemical and chemical studies of the localization of adrenergic and cholinergic nerves in novinal and denervated cat hearts. *Circulation Research*, **20**, 289–98.

James, T.N. & Sherf, L. (1968). Ultrastructure of the human atrioventricular node. *Circulation*, **37**, 1049–70.

James, T.N., Sherf, L., Fine, G. & Morales, A.R. (1966). Comparative ultrastructure of the sinus node in man and dog. *Circulation*, **34**, 139–63.

James, T.N., Sherf, L. & Urthaler, F. (1974). Fine structure of the bundle-branches. *British Heart Journal*, **36**, 1–18.

Jamieson, J.O. & Palade, G.E. (1964). Specific granules in atrial muscle cells. *Journal of Cell Biology*, **23**, 151–72.

Jynge, P., Hearse, D.J., de Leiris, J., Feuvray, D. & Braimbridge, M.V. (1978). Protection of the ischaemic myocardium: ultrastructural, enzymatic and functional assessment of various cardioplegic infusates. *Journal of Thoracic and Cardiovascular Surgery*, **76**, 2–15.

Kangawa, K. & Matsuo, H. (1984). Purification and complete amino acid sequence of human atrial natriuretic polypeptide (-hANP). *Biochemical and Biophysical Research Communications*, **118**, 131–9.

Kanno, Y. & Loewenstein, W. (1964). Intercellular diffusion. *Science*, **143**, 959–60.

Kappagoda, C.T., Knapp, M.F., Linden, R.J. & Whittaker, E.M. (1976). A possible bioassay for the humoral agent responsible for the diuresis from atrial receptors. *Journal of Physiology*, **254**, 59P.

Kappagoda, C.T., Linden, R.J. & Snow, H.M. (1972). The effect of distending the atrial appendages on urine flow in the dog. *Journal of Physiology*, **227**, 233–42.

Kaufman, M.H. & Navaratnam, V. (1981). Early differentiation of the heart in mouse embryos. *Journal of Anatomy*, **133**, 235–46.

Kawamura, K. & James, T.N. (1971). Comparative ultrastructure of cellular junctions in working myocardium and the conduction system under normal and pathologic conditions. *Journal of Molecular and Cellular Cardiology*, **3**, 31–60.

Kensler, R.W., Brink, P. & Dewey, M.M. (1977). Nexus of frog ventricle. *Journal of Cell Biology*, **73**, 768–81.

Kent, K.M., Epstein, S.E., Cooper, T. & Jacobowitz, D.M. (1974). Cholinergic innervation of the canine and human ventricular conducting system. Anatomic and electrophysiologic correlations. *Circulation Research*, **50**, 948–55.

Keynes, R.J., Smith, G.W., Slater, J.D.H., Brown, M.M., Brown, S.E., Payne, N.N., Jowett, T.P. & Monge, C.C. (1982). Renin and aldosterone at high altitude in man. *Journal of Endocrinology*, **92**, 131–40.

Kim, S. & Baba, N. (1971). Atrioventricular node and Purkinje fibers of the guinea-pig heart. *American Journal of Anatomy*, **132**, 339–54.

Kirklin, J.W. & Barratt-Boyes, B.G. (1986). *Cardiac Surgery*. New York: John Wiley.

Kisch, B. (1956). Electron microscopy of the atrium of the heart. *Experimental Medicine and Surgery*, **14**, 99–112.

Kisch, B. (1963a). A significant electron microscopic difference between the atria and ventricles of the mammalian heart. *Experimental Medicine and Surgery*, **21**, 193–221.

Kisch, B. (1963b). The perinuclear space in cardiac muscle (a spot of high enzyme activity). *Experimental Medicine and Surgery*, **21**, 222–30.

Kloner, R.A., De Boer, L.W.V., Darsee, J.R., Ingwall, J.S., Hale, S., Tumas, J. & Braunwald, E. (1981). Prolonged abnormalities of myocardium salvaged by reperfusion. *American Journal of Physiology*, **231**, H591–H599.

Kloner, R.A., Fishbein, M.C., Hare, C.M. & Maroko, P.R. (1979). Early ischaemic ultrastructural and histochemical alterations in the myocardium of the rat following coronary artery occlusion. *Experimental Molecular Pathology*, **30**, 129–43.

Knapp, M.F., Hicks, M.N., Linden, R.J. & Mary, D.A.S.G. (1986). Evidence against ANP as a natriuretic hormone during atrial distension. *Journal of Endocrinology*, **109**, R5–R8.

Kobayashi, Y., Hassall, C.J.S. & Burnstock, G. (1986a). Culture of intramural cardiac ganglia of the newborn guinea-pig. I. Neuronal elements. *Cell and Tissue Research* **244**, 595–604.

Kobayashi, Y., Hassall, C.J.S. & Burnstock, G. (1986b). Culture of intramural cardiac ganglia of the newborn guinea-pig. II. Non-neuronal elements. *Cell and Tissue Research* **244**, 605–12.

Kogon, M. & Pappas, G.D. (1976). Atypical gap junctions in the ciliary epithelium of the albino rabbit eye. *Journal of Cell Biology*, **66**, 671–6.

Konishi, S., Okamoto, T. & Otsuka, M. (1984). Synaptic transmission and effects of substance P and somatostatin on the guinea-pig cardiac ganglia. *IUPHAR Proceedings*, 1604.

Koobs, D.H., Schultz, R.L. & Jutzy, R.V. (1978). The origin of lipofuscin and possible consequences to the myocardium. *Archives of Pathology and Laboratory medicine*, **102**, 253–68.

Kordylewski, L., Goings, G., Karrison, K. & Page, E. (1985). Developmental changes in internal structure of chick heart plasma membrane. *Developmental Biology*, **112**, 485–8.

Kuhn, H., Richards, J.G. & Tranzer, J.P. (1975). The nature of rat 'specific heart granules' with regard to catecholamines: an investigation by ultrastructural cytochemistry. *Journal of Ultrastructure Research*, **50**, 159–66.

Lane, M-A., Sastre, A., Law, M. & Salpeter, M.M. (1977). Cholinergic and adrenergic receptors on mouse cardiocytes *in vitro*. *Developmental Biology*, **57**, 254–69.

Lane, N.J. & Swales, L.S. (1980). Dispersal of gap junctional particles not internalized during the in vivo disappearance of gap junctions. *Cell*, **19**, 579–86.

Lang, R.E., Thölken, H., Ganten, D., Luft, F.C., Ruskoaho, H. & Unger, T. (1985). Atrial natriuretic factor – a circulating hormone stimulated by volume loading. *Nature*, 314, 264–6.

Langer, G.A., Frank, J.S. & Philipson, K.D. (1982). Ultrastructure and calcium exchange of the sarcolemma, sarcoplasmic reticulum and mitochondria of the myocardium. *Pharmacology and Therapeutics*, 16, 331–76.

La Raia, P.J. & Sonnenblick, E.H. (1971). Autonomic control of cardiac c-AMP. *Circulation Research*, 28, 377–84.

Larsen, W.J. (1983). Biological implications of gap junction structure, distribution and composition: a review. *Tissue and Cell*, 15, 645–71.

Leader, F. (1963). Local cholinergic–adrenergic interaction: mechanism of the biphasic chronotropic response to nerve stimulation. *Journal of Pharmacology and Experimental Therapeutics*, 142, 31–8.

Lee, W.M., Cran, D.G. & Lane, N.J. (1982). Carbon dioxide induced disassembly of gap junctional plaques. *Journal of Cell Science*, 57, 214–28.

Leeson, T.S. (1980). Non-fibrillar filamentous material in right atrial myocardial cells of the rat. *Journal of Molecular and Cellular Cardiology*, 12, 267–84.

Legato, M.J. (1979). The ultrastructure of foetal dog myocardium. *Circulation*, Suppl. 60, II–44.

Leger, J.J., Bouveret, P., Schwartz, K. & Swynghedauw, B. (1976). A comparative study of skeletal and cardiac tropomyosins. *Pflügers Archiv European Journal of Physiology*, 362, 271–7.

Lemanski, L.F., Fitts, E.P. & Marx, B.S. (1975). Fine structure of the heart in the Japanese Medaka, *Oryzias latipes*. *Journal of Ultrastructure Research*, 53, 37–65.

Lever, J.D., Ahmed, M. & Irvine, G. (1965). Neuromuscular and intercellular relationships in the coronary arteries. A morphological and quantitative study by light and electron microscopy. *Journal of Anatomy*, 99, 829–40.

Levy, M.N. (1971). Sympathetic–parasympathetic interactions in the heart. *Circulation Research*, 29, 437–45.

Levy, M.N. & Zieske, H. (1969). Effect of enhanced contractility on the left ventricular response to vagus nerve stimulation in dogs. *Circulation Research*, 24, 303–11.

Lewis, P.R. & Knight, D.P. (1977). Staining methods for sectioned material. In *Practical Methods in Electron Microscopy*, vol. 5 (ed. A.M. Glauert). Amsterdam: North-Holland Publishing Company.

Lindal, S., Myklebust, R., Sørlie, D. & Jørgensen, L. (1983). Morphologic changes in atrial myocardial cells after cold cardioplegic standstill and during reperfusion in coronary bypass surgery. *Scandinavian Journal of Thoracic and Cardiovascular Surgery*, 17, 109–19.

Lindner, E. (1957). Die submikroskopische Morphologie des Herzmuskels. *Zeitschrift für Zellforschung und mikroskopische Anatomie*, 45, 702–46.

Lochner, A., Sanan, D., Victor, J., Bester, R., Kotze, J.C.N., Van der Merwe, N. & Schabort, I. (1986). Mitochondrial and sarcolemmal function and composition in myocardial ischaemia. *Journal of Molecular and Cellular Cardiology*, **18**, Suppl. 1, p. 344.

Loewenstein, W.R. (1981). Junctional intercellular communication: the cell-to-cell membrane channel. *Physiological Reviews*, **61**, 829–913.

Lolley, D.M., Ray, J.F. III, Myers, W.O., Sautter, R.D. & Tewksbury, D.A. (1979). Importance of preoperative myocardial glycogen levels in human cardiac preservation. *Journal of Thoracic and Cardiovascular Surgery*, **78**, 678–87.

Losman, J.G. (1980). Cardiac transplantation. In *Hearts and Heart-like Organs*, vol. 3 (ed. G.H. Bourne), pp. 349–414. New York: Academic Press.

Luft, J.H. (1971). Ruthenium red and violet. II. Fine structural localization in animal tissues. *Anatomical Record*, **171**, 369–416.

Lüllman, H., Peters, T. & Preuner, J. (1983). Role of the plasmalemma for calcium homeostasis and for excitation-contraction coupling in cardiac muscle. In *Cardiac Metabolism* (ed. A.J. Drake-Holland. & M.I.M. Noble), pp. 1–18. Chichester: John Wiley. & Sons.

Lyman, C.P., O'Brien, R.C. & Green, G.C. (1981). Hibernation and longevity in the Turkish hamster *Mesocricetus brandti*. *Science*, **212**, 668–70.

Makowski, L., Caspar, D.L.D., Phillips, W.C. & Goodenough, D.A. (1977). Gap junction structures. II. Analysis of the X-ray diffraction data. *Journal of Cell Biology*, **74**, 629–95.

Malkoff, D.B. & Strehler, B.L. (1963). The ultrastructure of isolated and in situ human cardiac age pigment. *Journal of Cell Biology*, **16**, 611–16.

Malor, R., Taylor, S., Chesher, G.B. & Griffin, C.J. (1974). The intramural ganglia and chromaffin cells in guinea pig atria: an ultrastructural study. *Cardiovascular Research*, **8**, 731–44.

Malouf, N.N. & Meissner, G. (1984). Methods for histochemical localization of surface membrane 'basic' ATPase and sarcoplasmic reticulum $(Ca^{2+} + Mg^{2+})$ ATPase in heart. In *Methods in Studying Cardiac Membranes*, vol. 2 (ed. N.S. Dhalla), pp. 99–109. Boca Raton, Florida: C.R.C. Press.

Manasek, F.J. (1969). Embryonic development of the heart. II. Formation of the epicardium. *Journal of Embryology and Experimental Morphology*, **22**, 333–48.

Manasek, F.J. (1976). Heart development: interactions involved in cardiac morphogenesis. In *The Cell Surface in Animal Embryogenesis and Development* (ed. G. Poste & G.L. Nicholson), pp. 545–98. Amsterdam: North-Holland Publishing Co.

Manning, P., Schwartz, D., Katsube, N.C., Holmberg, S.W. & Needleman, P. (1985). Vasopressin-stimulated release of atriopeptin: endocrine antagonists in fluid homeostasis. *Science*, **229**, 395–7.

Martinez-Palomo, A. & Alanis, J. (1980). The amphibian and reptile hearts: Impulse propagation and ultrastructure. In *Hearts and Heartlike Organs*, vol. 1 (ed. G.H. Bourne), pp. 171–97. New York: Academic Press.

Martinez-Palomo, A. & Mendez, R. (1971). Presence of gap junctions between cardiac cells in the heart of nonmammalian species. *Journal of Ultrastructure Research*, 37, 592–600.

Masters, T.N. & Glaviano, V.V. (1972). The effects of norepinephrine and propranolol on myocardial subcellular distribution of triglycerides and free fatty acids. *Journal of Pharmacology and Experimental Therapeutics*, 182, 246–55.

Mazet, F. (1977). Freeze-fracture studies of gap junctions in the developing and adult amphibian cardiac muscle. *Developmental Biology*, 60, 139–52.

Mazet, F. (1985). Filipin/Digitonin studies of membrane cholesterol in frog atrial fibres with the unusual gap junction configuration. *European Journal of Cell Biology*, 36, Suppl. 8, p. 19.

Mazet, F. & Cartaud, J. (1976). Freeze-fracture studies of frog atrial fibres. *Journal of Cell Science*, 22, 427–34.

Mazet, F., Wittenberg, B.A. & Spray, D.C. (1985). Fate of intercellular junctions in isolated adult rat cardiac cells. *Circulation Research*, 56, 194–204.

McCallister, L.P., Daiello, D.C. & Tyers, G.F.O. (1978). Morphometric observations of the effects of normothermic ischemic arrest on dog myocardial ultrastructure. *Journal of Molecular and Cellular Cardiology*, 10, 67–80.

McKenzie, J.C., Tanaka, I., Misono, K.S. & Inagami, T. (1985). Immunocytochemical localization of atrial natriuretic factor in the kidney, adrenal medulla, pituitary and atrium of rat. *Journal of Histochemistry and Cytochemistry*, 33, 828–32.

McMahan, V.J. & Purves, D. (1976). Visual identification of two kinds of nerve cells and their synaptic contacts in a living autonomic ganglion of the mud puppy (*Necturus maculosus*). *Journal of Physiology*, 254, 405–25.

McNutt, N.S. (1975). Ultrastructure of the myocardial sarcolemma. *Circulation Research*, 37, 1–13.

McNutt, N.S. & Weinstein, R.S. (1970). The ultrastructure of the nexus. *Journal of Cell Biology*, 47, 666–88.

Melax, H. & Leeson, T.S. (1970). Fine structure of the impulse-conducting system in rat heart. *Canadian Journal of Zoology*, 48, 837–9.

Menz, L.J., Kolata, R.J., Standeven, J.W., Codd, J.E. & Miller, L.W. (1984). Study of orthotopic transplanted dog hearts stored or perfused hypothermically: ultrastructure *vs* haemodynamic performance. *Cryobiology*, 21, 702–3.

Michalke, W. & Loewenstein, W. (1971). Communication between cells of different types. *Nature*, 232, 121–2.

Mitchell, G.A.G., Brown, R. & Cookson, F. (1953). Ventricular nerve cells in mammals. *Nature*, 172, 812.

Mochet, M., Moravec, J., Guillemot, H. & Hatt, P.Y. (1975). The ultrastructure of rat conductive tissue: an electron microscopic study of the atrioventricular node and the bundle of His. *Journal of Molecular and Cellular Cardiology*, 7, 879–89.

Moore, D.H. & Ruska, H. (1957). The fine structure of capillaries and small arteries. *Journal of Biophysical and Biochemical Cytology*, 3, 457–62.

Morgan, J., Bittner, S. & Cohen, L. (1978). Calcium protection of myocardium: ultrastructural studies. *Federation Proceedings*, 37, 899.

Muir, A.R. (1957). Observations on the fine structure of the Purkinje fibres of the sheep's heart. *Journal of Anatomy*, 91, 251–8.

Müller, P. (1966). Lokale Kontraktionsauslösung am Herzmuskel. *Helvetica physiologica et pharmacologica Acta*, 24, C106–C108.

Nandy, K. & Bourne, G.H. (1963). A study of the morphology of the conducting tissue in mammalian hearts. *Acta anatomica*, 53, 217–26.

Nathanson, N.M. (1983). Binding of agonists and antagonists to muscarinic acetylcholine receptors on intact cultured heart cells. *Journal of Neurochemistry*, 41, 1545–9.

Natori, R. (1975). The electric potential change of internal membrane during propagation of contraction in skinned fibre of toad skeletal muscle. *Japanese Journal of Physiology*, 25, 51–63.

Navaratnam, V. (1965a). The ontogenesis of cholinesterase activity within the heart and cardiac ganglia in man, rat, rabbit and guinea-pig. *Journal of Anatomy*, 99, 459–67.

Navaratnam, V. (1965b). Development of the nerve supply to the mammalian heart. *British Heart Journal*, 27, 640–50.

Navaratnam, V. (1978). The structure of cardiac muscle. In *Developments in Cardiovascular Medicine* (ed. C.J. Dickinson & J. Marks), pp. 119–28. Lancaster: MTP Press.

Navaratnam, V. (1980). Anatomy of the mammalian heart. In *Hearts and Heart-like Organs*, vol. 1 (ed. G.H. Bourne), pp. 349–74. New York: Academic Press.

Navaratnam, V., Ayettey, A.S., Addae, F., Kesse, K. & Skepper, J.N. (1986a). Ultrastructure of the ventricular myocardium of the bat *Eidolon helvum*. *Acta anatomica*, 126, 240–3.

Navaratnam, V., Kaufman, M.H., Skepper, J.N., Barton, S. & Guttridge, K.M. (1986b). Differentiation of the myocardial rudiment in mouse embryos: an ultrastructural study including freeze-fracture replication. *Journal of Anatomy*, 146, 65–85.

Navaratnam, V., Lewis, P.R. & Shute, C.C.D. (1968). Effects of vagotomy on the cholinesterase content of the preganglionic innervation of the rat heart. *Journal of Anatomy*, 103, 225–32.

Navaratnam, V. & Palkama, A. (1965). Cholinesterases in the walls of the great arterial trunks and coronary arteries. *Acta anatomica*, 63, 445–8.

Navaratnam, V., Skepper, J.N. & Thurley, K.W. (1980). Freeze-fracture studies using melting nitrogen slush as quenching medium. *Journal of Anatomy*, 131, 776.

Navaratnam, V., Thurley, K.W. & Skepper, J.N. (1982). Freeze-fracture replication studies of mammalian heart muscle. In *Progress in Anatomy*, vol. 2 (ed. R.J. Harrison & V. Navaratnam), pp. 201–15. Cambridge: Cambridge University Press.

Nayler, W.G., Gran, A. & Yepez, C. (1978). Pharmacologic protection of hypoxic hearts. In *Recent Advances in Studies on Cardiac Structure and Metabolism*, vol. 12 (ed. T. Kobayashi, Y. Ito & G. Rona), pp. 525–30. Baltimore: University Park Press.

Nayler, W.G. & Merrillees, N.C.R. (1971). Cellular exchange of calcium. In *Calcium and the Heart* (ed. P. Harris & L. Opie), pp. 24–65. London: Academic Press.

Needleman, P. (1986). Atriopeptin biochemical pharmacology. *Federation Proceedings*, **45**, 2096–100.

Nelson, D.A. & Benson, E.S. (1963). On the structural continuities of the transverse tubular system of rabbit and human myocardial cells. *Journal of Cell Biology*, **16**, 297–313.

Nicholson, B.J., Takemoto, L.J., Hunkapiller, M.W., Hood, L.E. & Revel, J-P. (1983). Differences between liver gap junction protein and lens MIP 26 from rat: implications for tissue specificity of gap junctions. *Cell*, **32**, 967–78.

Nielsen, K.C. & Owman, C.H. (1968). Difference in cardiac adrenergic innervation between hibernators and non-hibernating mammals. *Acta physiologica Scandinavica*, **316**, 1–30.

Noble, D. (1975). *The Initiation of the Heartbeat*. Oxford: Clarendon Press.

Noble, M.I.M. (1983). Excitation-contraction coupling. In *Cardiac Metabolism* (ed. A.J. Drake-Holland & M.I.M. Noble), pp. 49–71. Chichester: John Wiley & Sons.

Nonidez, J.F. (1939). Studies on the innervation of the heart. *American Journal of Anatomy*, **65**, 361–413.

Nonoyama, A., Kasahara, K., Fukunaka, M., Sato, T., Masuda, A., Kotani, A. & Kagawa, T. (1978). Myocardial protection during open heart surgery: preservation of myocardial metabolism and ultrastructure by cold coronary perfusion. In *Recent Advances in Studies on Cardiac Structure and Metabolism*, vol. 12 (ed. T. Kobayashi, Y. Ito & G. Rona), pp. 479–84. Baltimore: University Park Press.

Norberg, K-A. & Sjoqvist, P. (1966). New possibilities for adrenergic modulation of ganglionic transmission. *Pharmacological Reviews*, **18**, 743–51.

Novi, A.M. (1968). An electron microscopic study of the innervation of papillary muscles in the rat. *Anatomical Record*, **160**, 123–42.

Novikoff, A.B. (1963). Lysosomes in the physiology and pathology of cells: contributions of staining methods. In *CIBA Foundation Symposium on Lysosomes* (ed. A.V.S. de Reuch & M.P. Cameron Little), pp. 36–73. Boston: Brown & Co.

Novikoff, A.B. (1964). GERL, its formation and functions in neurons of rat spinal ganglia. *Biological Bulletins*, **127**, 358-A.

Novikoff, A.B., Essner, E. & Quintana, N. (1964). Golgi apparatus and lysosomes. *Federation Proceedings*, **23**, 1010–22.

Novikoff, P.M., Novikoff, A.B., Quintana, N. & Hauw, J-J. (1971). Golgi apparatus, GERL and lysosomes of neurons in rat dorsal root ganglia studied by thick section and thin section cytochemistry. *Journal of Cell Biology*, **50**, 859–86.

Ogawa, K. & Mayohara, H. (1969). Intramitochondrial localisation of adenosine triphosphatase activity. *Journal of Histochemistry and Cytochemistry*, **17**, 487–90.

Olson, L., Ålund, M. & Norberg, K-A. (1976). Fluorescence microscopical demonstration of a population of gastrointestinal nerve fibres with a selective affinity for quinacrine. *Cell and Tissue Research*, **171**, 407–23.

Opie, L.H. (1968). Metabolism of the heart in health and disease, Part I. *American Heart Journal*, **76**, 685–98.

Opie, L.H., Owen, P. & Riemersma, R.S. (1973). Relative rates of oxidation of glucose and free fatty acids by ischaemic and non-ischaemic myocardium after coronary artery ligation in the dog. *European Journal of Clinical Investigation*, **3**, 419–35.

Øskendal, A., Jynge, P., Greve, G. & Saetersdal, T. (1984). Tissue protection by verapamil in the calcium paradox. *Journal of Molecular and Cellular Cardiology*, **16**, Suppl. 2, p. 20.

Otsuka, N., Okamoto, H. & Tomisawa, M. (1969). Electron and fluorescence microscopic study of specific granules in rat atrial muscle cells. *Archives of Histology, Japan*, **30**, 367–74.

Page, E. (1967*a*). Tubular systems in Purkinje cells of the cat heart. *Journal of Ultrastructure Research*, **17**, 72–83.

Page, E. (1967*b*). The occurrence of inclusions within membrane-limited structures that run longitudinally in the cells of mammalian heart muscle. *Journal of Ultrastructure Research*, **17**, 63–71.

Page, E. (1968). Correlations between electron microscopic and physiological observations in heart muscle. *Journal of General Physiology*, **51**, 211–20.

Page, E. & Manjunath, C.K. (1985). Biochemistry and structure of cardiac gap junctions: recent observations. In *Gap Junctions* (ed. M.V.L. Bennett & D.C. Spray), pp. 49–56. Cold Spring Harbor Laboratory.

Palade, G.E. (1961). Secretory granules in the atrial myocardium. *Anatomical Record*, **139**, 262.

Papafrangas, E.D. & Lyman, C.P. (1982). Lipofuscin accumulation and hibernation in the Turkish hamster *Mesocricetus brandti*. *Journal of Gerontology*, **37**, 417–21.

Papka, R.E. (1974). A study of catecholamine-containing cells in the hearts of foetal and postnatal rabbits by fluorescence and electron microscopy. *Cell and Tissue Research*, **154**, 471–84.

Papka, R.E. (1976). Studies of cardiac ganglia in pre- and postnatal rabbits. *Cell and Tissue Research*, **175**, 17–35.

Parker, F. (1958). Electron microscopical study of coronary arteries. *American Journal of Anatomy*, **103**, 247–73.

Patten, B.M. & Kramer, T.C. (1933). The initiation of contraction in the embryonic chick heart. *American Journal of Anatomy*, **53**, 349–75.

Peachey, L.D., Waugh, R.A. & Sommer, J.R. (1974). High voltage electron microscopy of sarcoplasmic reticulum. *Journal of Cell Biology*, **63**, 262a.

Pearce, J.W. & Sonnenberg, H. (1965). Effects of spinal section and renal denervation on renal response to blood volume expansion. *Canadian Journal of Physiology and Pharmacology*, **43**, 211–24.

Perlmutt, J.H., Aziz, O. & Haberich, F.J. (1975). A comparison of sodium excretion in response to infusion of isotonic saline into the vena porta and vena cava of conscious rats. *Pflüger's Archiv*, **357**, 1–14.

Perman, E. (1924). Anatomische Untersuchungen uber die Herznerven bei den hoheren Saugetieren und beim Menschen. *Zeitschrift für Anatomie und Entwicklungsgeschichte*, **71**, 382–457.

Perracchia, C. & Girsch, S.J. (1985). Functional modulation of cell coupling; evidence for a calmodulin-driven channel. *American Journal of Physiology*, **248**, H765–H782.

Peters, A., Palay, S.L. & Webster, H.F. (1970). *The Fine Structure of the Nervous System; the Cells and Their Processes*. London: Harper & Row.

Peterson, T.V., Felts, F.T. & Chase, N.L. (1983). Intravascular receptors and renal responses of monkey to volume expansion. *American Journal of Physiology*, **244**, H55–H59.

Pomerance, A. (1976). Pathology of the myocardium and valves. In *Cardiology in Old Age*, chapter 2 (ed. F.I. Caird, J.L.C. Dall & R.D. Kennedy), pp. 11–55. New York: Plenum Press.

Pricam, C., Humbert, F., Perrelet, A. & Orci, L. (1974). Gap junctions in mesangial and lacis cells. *Journal of Cell Biology*, **63**, 349–54.

Prickaerts, J.P., Wilson, J.P., Bayliss, C.E. & Baffour, R. (1984). Influence of fixative osmolality on the morphometric determination of extracellular space in normal and reperfused myocardium. *Journal of Microscopy*, **135**, 169–79.

Prinzen, F.W. (1982). Gradients in blood flow, mechanics and metabolism in the ischemic left ventricular wall of the dog. *Thesis*, University of Limburg, The Netherlands.

Priola, D.V. & Fulton, R.L. (1969). Positive and negative responses of the atria and ventrioles to vagosympathetic stimulation in the isovolumic canine heart. *Circulation Research*, **25**, 265–75.

Randall, W.C., Priola, D.V. & Pace, J.B. (1967). Responses of individual cardiac chambers to stimulation of the cervical vagosympathetic trunk in atropinised dogs. *Circulation Research*, **20**, 534–44.

Raviola, E. & Gilula, N.B. (1973). Gap junctions between photoreceptor cells in the vertebrate retina. *Proceedings of the National Academy of Science, U.S.A.*, **70**, 1677–81.

Rayns, D.G., Devine, C.E. & Sutherland, C.L. (1975). Freeze fracture studies of membrane systems in vertebrate muscle. I. Striated muscle. *Journal of Ultrastructure Research*, **50**, 306–21.

Rayns, D.G., Simpson, F.O. & Bertaud, W.S. (1968). Surface features of striated muscle. I. Guinea pig cardiac muscle. *Journal of Cell Science*, **3**, 467–74.

Revel, J.P. & Karnovsky, M.J. (1967). Hexagonal array of subunits in intercellular junctions of the mouse heart and liver. *Journal of Cell Biology*, **33**, C7–C12.

Revel, J.P., Yee, A.G. & Hudspeth, A.J. (1971). Gap junctions between electronically coupled cells in tissue culture and in brown fat. *Proceedings of the National Academy of Science, U.S.A.*, **68**, 2924–7.

Robinek, H., Jung, H. & Gebhard, R. (1982). The topography of filipin-cholesterol complexes in the plasma membrane of cultured hepatocytes and their relationship to cell junction formation. *Journal of Ultrastructure Research*, **78**, 95–106.

Robinson, J.M. & Karnovsky, M.J. (1983). Ultrastructural localization of several phosphatases with cerium. *Journal of Histochemistry and Cytochemistry*, **31**, 1197–208.

Roper, S. (1976). An electrophysiological study of chemical and electrical synapses on neurones in the parasympathetic cardiac ganglion of the mud puppy, *Necturus maculosus*: evidence for intrinsic ganglion innervation. *Journal of Physiology*, **254**, 427–54.

Rosenquist, G.C. & De Haan, R.L. (1966). Migration of pericardiac cells in the embryonic chick heart. *American Journal of Anatomy*, **53**, 349–75.

Rossi, L. & Bassi, M. (1962). Le sous-endocarde gauche du septum ventriculaire chez le cobaye. Étude au microscope électronique. *Archives des Maladies du Coeur et des Vaisseaux*, **55**, 919–25.

Ruigrok, T.J.C., Slade, A-M., van der Meer, P., De Moes, D., Sinclair, D.M., Poole-Wilson, P.A. & Meijler, F.L. (1985). Different effects of thiopental in severe hypoxia, total ischemia and low-flow ischemia in rat heart muscle. *Anesthesiology*, **63**, 172–8.

Sabin, F.R. (1920). Studies on the origin of blood vessels and of red blood corpuscles as seen in the living blastoderm of chicks during the second day of incubation. *Contributions to Embryology*, **9**, 213–62.

Sachs, H.G., Colgan, J.H. & Lazarus, M.L. (1977). Ultrastructure of the aging myocardium: a morphometric approach. *American Journal of Anatomy*, **150**, 63–72.

Samarajski, T., Ordy, J.M. & Keefe, J.R. (1965). The fine structure of lipofuscin age pigment in the nervous system of aged mice. *Journal of Cell Biology*, **26**, 779–95.

Samarajski, T., Ordy, J.M. & Rady-Reimer, P. (1968). Lipofuscin pigment accumulation in the nervous system of aging mice. *Anatomical Record*, **160**, 555–74.

Sanan, D.A., van der Merwe, E.L. & Lochner, A. (1985). Comparison of the effects of immersion and perfusion fixation on the ultrastructure of mitochondria from severely ischaemic myocardium. *South African Journal of Science*, **81**, 564–70.

Sandborn, E.B., Côté, M.G., Roberge, J. & Bois, P. (1967). Microtubules et filaments cytoplasmiques dans le muscle de mammifères. *Journal de Microscopie*, **6**, 169–78.

Santer, R.M. (1985). Morphology and innervation of the fish heart. In *Advances in Anatomy, Embryology and Cell Biology*, vol. 89. Berlin: Springer-Verlag.

Sarnoff, S.J., Brockman, S.K., Gilmore, J.P., Linden, R.J. & Mitchell, J.H.

(1960). Regulation of ventricular contraction: influence of cardiac sympathetic and vagal stimulation on atrial and ventricular dynamics. *Circulation Research*, 8, 1108–22.

Sashida, H. & Abiko, Y. (1986). Protective effect of Diltiazem on ultrastructural alterations induced by coronary occlusion and reperfusion in dog hearts. *Journal of Molecular and Cellular Cardiology*, 18, 401–11.

Schaffer, S.W., Burton, K.P., Jones, H.P. & Oei, H.H. (1983). Phenothiazine protection in calcium overload-induced heart failure: a possible role for calmodulin. *American Journal of Physiology*, 244, H328–H334.

Schaper, J., Meiser, E. & Stämmler, G. (1985). Ultrastructural morphometric analysis of myocardium from dogs, rats, hamsters, mice, and from human hearts. *Circulation Research*, 56, 377–91.

Schaper, J., Stämmler, G. & Scheld, H. (1981). The effects of global ischemia and reperfusion on human myocardium: quantitative evaluation by electron microscopic morphometry. *Annals of Thoracic Surgery*, 33, 116–22.

Schaper, T., Pinkowski, E. & Froede, R. (1982). Ultrastructural changes of mitochondria in ischemic and reperfused canine myocardium. *Journal of Molecular and Cellular Cardiology*, 14, Suppl. 1, p. 59.

Schenk, E.A. & El Badawi, A. (1968). Dual innervation of arteries and arterioles. A histochemical study. *Zeitschrift für Zellforschung und mikroskopische Anatomie*, 91, 170–7.

Scheuermann, D.W. & De Maziere, A. (1984). Gap junctions in the heart of the adult *Protopterus aethiopicus*. *Acta Morphologica Neerlando-Scandinavica*, 22, 123–31.

Schiebler, T.H. (1955). Herzstudie. II. Mitteilung. Histologische, histochemische und experimetelle Untersuchungen am Atrioventrikularsystem von Huf- und Nagetieren. *Zeitschrift für Zellforschung und microskopische Anatomie*, 43, 243–306.

Schultze, W. (1984). Methods for histochemical localization of adenylate cyclase and guanylate cyclase in heart membranes. In *Methods in Studying Cardiac Membranes*, vol. 2 (ed. N.S. Dhalla), pp. 83–97. Boca Raton, Florida: C.R.C. Press.

Schvalev, V.N. & Sosunov, A.A. (1985). A light and electron microscopic study of cardiac ganglia in mammals. *Zeitschrift für anatomische Forschung*, 99, 676–94.

Severs, N.J. (1984). Freeze-fracture cytochemical methods for studying the distribution of cholesterol in heart membranes. In *Methods in Studying Cardiac Membranes*, vol. 2 (ed. N.S. Dhalla), pp. 27–44. Boca Raton, Florida: C.R.C. Press.

Sheridan, D.J., Cullen, M.J. & Tynan, M.J. (1979). Postnatal ultrastructural changes in the cat myocardium: a morphometric study. *Cardiovascular Research*, 11, 536–40.

Shibata, Y., Nakata, K. & Page, E. (1980). Ultrastructural changes during development of gap junctions in rabbit left ventricular myocardial cells. *Journal of Ultrastructure Research*, 71, 258–71.

Shibata, Y. & Page, E. (1981). Gap junctional structure in intact and cut sheep cardiac purkinje fibres: a freeze-fracture study of Ca^{2+}-induced resealing. *Journal of Ultrastructure Research*, **75**, 195–204.

Shibata, Y. & Yamamoto, T. (1979). Freeze-fracture studies of gap junctions in vertebrate cardiac muscle cells. *Journal of Ultrastructure Research*, **67**, 79–88.

Shiraishi, Y., Chiba, Y., Tatsuta, N., Hikasa, Y. & Suzusho, T. (1980). Experimental study of myocardial protection of cold blood cardioplegia: ultrastructure of ischemic myocardium. *Journal of Clinical Electron Microscopy*, **13**, 747–8.

Simpson, F.O. (1965). The transverse tubular system in mammalian myocardial cells. *American Journal of Anatomy*, **117**, 1–18.

Simpson, F.O. & Oertalis, S.J. (1961). Relationship of the sarcolemma in sheep cardiac muscle. *Nature*, **189**, 758–9.

Simpson, F.R. & Oertalis, S.J. (1962). The fine structure of sheep myocardial cells: sarcolemmal invaginations and the transverse tubular system. *Journal of Cell Biology*, **12**, 91–100.

Simpson, F.O., Rayns, D.G. & Ledingham, J.M. (1973). The ultrastructure of ventricular and atrial myocardium. In *Ultrastructure of the Mammalian Heart* (ed. C.E. Challice & S. Virágh), pp. 1–41. New York: Academic Press.

Sissman, N.J. (1970). Developmental landmarks in cardiac morphogenesis: comparative chronology. *American Journal of Cardiology*, **25**, 141–8.

Sjöstrand, F.S. & Andersson, E. (1954). Electron microscopy of the intercalated discs of cardiac muscle tissue. *Experientia*, **10**, 369–70.

Sjöstrand, F.S., Andersson-Cerdergren, E. & Dewey, M.M. (1958). The ultrastructure of the intercalated disc of frog, mouse and guinea pig cardiac muscle. *Journal of Ultrastructural Research*, **1**, 271–87.

Skepper, J.N. & Navaratnam, V. (1986). Variations in the structure of nexuses in the myocardium of the golden hamster *Mesocricetus auratus*. *Journal of Anatomy*, **149**, 143–55.

Skepper, J.N. & Navaratnam, V. (1987). Lipofuscin formation in juvenile golden hamsters: an ultrastructural study including staining for acid phosphatase. *Journal of Anatomy*, **150**, 155–67.

Skepper, J.N., Thurley, K.W. & Navaratnam, V. (1982). Specialised cell junctions in the nodal musculature of hamster and rat hearts. *Journal of Anatomy*, **135**, 836–7.

Slade, A.M. & Nayler, W.G. (1981). Effect of verapamil pretreatment on ischaemic and reperfused heart muscle: a morphometric study. *Journal of Molecular and Cellular Cardiology*, **13**, Suppl. 1, p. 88.

Smith, D.S., Baerwald, R.J. & Hart, M.A. (1975). The distribution of orthogonal assemblies and other intercalated particles in frog sartorius and rabbit sacrospinalis muscle. *Tissue and Cell*, **7**, 369–82.

Smith, H. (1957). Salt and water receptors. *American Journal of Medicine*, **23**, 623–52.

Smith, R.B. (1971). The occurrence and location of intrinsic cardiac ganglia and nerve plexuses in the human neonate. *Anatomical Record*, **169**, 33–40.

Smith, R.E. & Farquhar, M.G. (1966). Lysosome formation in the regulation of the secretory process in cells of the anterior pituitary gland. *Journal of Cell Biology*, **31**, 319–47.

Sommer, J.R. (1982). Ultrastructural considerations concerning cardiac muscle. *Journal of Molecular and Cellular Cardiology*, **14**, Suppl. 3, pp. 77–83.

Sommer, J.R. & Johnson, E.A. (1968a). Cardiac muscle. A comparative study of Purkinje fibers and ventricular fibers. *Journal of Cell Biology*, **36**, 497–526.

Sommer, J.R. & Johnson, E.A. (1986b). Purkinje fibers of the heart examined with the peroxidase reaction. *Journal of Cell Biology*, **37**, 570–4.

Sommer, J.R. & Johnson, E.A. (1969). Cardiac muscle. A comparative ultrastructure study with special reference to frog and chicken. *Zeitschrift für Zellforschung un mikroskopische Anatomie*, **98**, 437–68.

Sommer, J.R. & Johnson, E.A. (1979). Ultrastructure of cardiac muscle. In *Handbook of Physiology*, section 2, vol. 1 (ed. R.M. Berne), chapter 5, pp. 113–86. Bethesda: American Physiological Society.

Sommer, J.R. & Spach, M.S. (1964). Electron microscopic demonstration of adenosine triphosphate in myofibrils and sarcoplasmic membranes of cardiac muscle of normal and abnormal dogs. *American Journal of Pathology*, **44**, 491–505.

Sonnenberg, H. (1985). Mechanisms of release and renal tubular action of atrial natriuretic factor. *Federation Proceedings*, **45**, 2106–10.

Sonnenblick, E.H., Ross Jr, J., Covell, J.W., Spotnitz, H.M. & Spiro, D. (1967). The ultrastructure of the heart in systole and diastole; changes in sarcomere length. *Circulation Research*, **21**, 423–31.

Sosa-Lucero, J.C., del le Iglesia, F.A., Lumb, G., Berger, J.M. & Bencosme, S. (1969). Subcellular distribution of catecholamines and specific granules in the rat heart. *Laboratory Investigations*, **21**, 19–26.

Spector, W.S. (1956). *Handbook of Biological Data*. Philadelphia: W.B. Saunders.

Sperelakis, N. & Mann, J.J.E., Jr. (1977). Evaluation of electric field changes in the clefts between excitable cells. *Journal of Theoretical Biology*, **64**, 71–96.

Sperelakis, N., Mayer, G. & Macdonald, R. (1970). Velocity of propagation in vertebrate cardiac muscles as functions of tonicity and $[K^+]o$. *American Journal of Physiology*, **219**, 952–63.

Spiro, D. & Sonnenblick, E.H. (1964). Comparison of the ultrastructural basis of the contractile process in heart and skeletal muscle. *Circulation Research*, **14–15**, Suppl. II, II.14–II.37.

Spoerri, P.E. & Glees, P. (1973). Neuronal aging in cultures: an electron-microscopic study. *Experimental Gerontology*, **8**, 259–63.

Spoerri, P.E. & Glees, P. (1974). The effects of dimethylaminoethyl *p*-chlorophenoxyacetate on spinal ganglia neurons and satellite cells in culture. Mitochondrial changes in the aging neurons. An electron microscope study. *Mechanisms of Ageing and Development*, **3**, 131–55.

Staehelin, L.A. (1974). Structure and function of intercellular junctions. *International Review of Cytology*, **39**, 191–283.

Staley, N.A. & Benson, E.S. (1968). The ultrastructure of frog ventricular cardiac muscle and its relationship to mechanisms of excitation-contraction coupling. *Journal of Cell Biology*, **38**, 99–114.

Standaert, D.G., Saper, C.B. & Needleman, P. (1985). Atriopeptin: potent hormone and potential neuromediator. *Trends in Neurosciences*, **8**, 509–11.

Stein, O. & Stein, Y. (1971). Light and electron microscopic autoradiography of lipids. Techniques and biological applications. *Advances in Lipid Research*, **9**, 1–72.

Strehler, B.L., Mark, D.D., Mildban, A.S. & Gee, M.V. (1959). Rate and magnitude of age pigment accumulation in the human myocardium. *Journal of Gerontology*, **14**, 430–9.

Sunamori, M., Hatano, R., Suzuki, T., Yamamoto, N., Tsukuhara, T., Yamada, T., Kumazawa, T., Nakagawa, M. & Sunaga, T. (1978). Ultrastructural change in myocardium subsequent to ischemic cardioplegia: 'no-reflow phenomenon'. In *Recent Advances in Studies on Cardiac Structure and Metabolism*, vol. 12 (ed. T. Kobayashi, Y. Ito & G. Rona), pp. 597–601. Baltimore: University Park Press.

Syska, H., Perry, S.V. & Trayer, I.P. (1974). A new method of preparation of troponin I (inhibitory protein) using affinity chromatography. Evidence for three different forms of troponin I in striated muscle. *Federation of European Biochemical Societies Letters*, **40**, 253–7.

Takayanagi, R., Tanaka, I., Maki, M. & Inagami, T. (1985). Effects of changes in water-sodium balance on levels of atrial natriuretic factor messenger RNA and peptide in rats. *Life Sciences*, **36**, 1843–8.

Takimoto, M., Matsuoka, S., Hirohata, T., Suzuki, Y., Enomoto, K., Ohta, H. & Okada, N. (1983). Myocardial protection during cardiac ischaemia by coronary perfusion with cold lactated Ringer's solution plus mannitol. *Japanese Heart Journal*, **24**, 199–214.

Tate, E.L. & Herbener, G.H. (1976). A morphometric study of the density of mitochondrial cristae in heart and liver of aging mice. *Journal of Gerontology*, **31**, 129–34.

Tay, S.S.W., Wong, W.C. & Ling, E.A. (1983). An ultrastructural study of small granule-containing cells in the heart of the monkey (*Macaca fascicularis*). *Journal of Anatomy*, **136**, 35–45.

Tay, S.S.W., Wong, W.C. & Ling, E.A. (1984a). An ultrastructural study of the neuronal changes in the cardiac ganglia of the monkey (*Macaca fascicularis*) following unilateral vagotomy. *Journal of Anatomy*, **138**, 67–80.

Tay, S.S.W., Wong, W.C. & Ling, E.A. (1984b). An ultrastructural study of the non-neuronal cells in the cardiac ganglia of the monkey (*Macaca fascicularis*) following unilateral vagotomy. *Journal of Anatomy*, **138**, 411–22.

Taylor, I.M. (1980). Observations on the sinuatrial nodal artery of the rat. *Journal of Anatomy*, **130**, 821–31.

Taylor, I.M. & Smith, R.B. (1971). Visualization of cholinesterase activity in the heart and lungs of the human foetus. *Journal of Anatomy*, **108**, 594–5.

Thaemert, J.C. (1973). Fine structure of the atrioventricular node as viewed in serial sections. *Anatomical Record*, **163**, 575–86.

Theron, J.J, Biagio, R., Meyer, A.C. & Boekkoi, S. (1978). Ultrastructural observations on the maturation and secretion of granules in atrial myocardium. *Journal of Molecular and Cellular Cardiology*, **10**, 567–72.

Thibault, G., Garcia, R., Cantin, M. & Genest, J. (1983). Atrial natriuretic factor. Characterization and partial purification. *Hypertension*, **5**, Suppl. 1, pp. 175–80.

Tice, L.W. & Barnett, R.J. (1962). Fine structural localization of adenosinetriphosphatase activity in heart muscle myofibrils. *Journal of Cell Biology*, **15**, 401–16.

Tomanek, R.J. & Karlsson, U.L. (1972). Myocardial ultrastructure of young and senescent rats. *Journal of Ultrastructure Research*, **40**, 201–20.

Tomisawa, M. (1969). Atrial specific granules in various mammals. *Archives of Histology, Japan*, **30**, 449–65.

Torok, B., Trombitás, K. & Röth, E. (1983). Ultrastructural consequences of reperfusion of the ischaemic myocardium. *Acta Morphologica Hungarica*, **31**, 315–26.

Travis, D.F. & Travis, A. (1972). Ultrastructural changes in the left ventricular rat myocardial cells with age. *Journal of Ultrastructure Research*, **39**, 124–48.

Uchida, H., Nakamura, M., Nakano, T., Takezawa, H., Yuasa, H. & Kusagawa, M. (1980). Electron microscopic changes of the myocardium before and after aortic cross clamping. *Journal of Clinical Electron Microscopy*, **13**, 746.

Uchizono, K. (1964). Innervation of the blood capillary in the heart of the dog and rabbit. *Japanese Journal of Physiology*, **14**, 587–98.

Ungar, R. (1924). Zür Anatomie der specifischen Muskelsystems im Menschenherzen. *Lotos*, **72**, 209–38.

Unwin, P.N.T. & Zampighi, G. (1980). Structure of the junctions between communicating cells. *Nature*, **283**, 545–9.

van Breemen, V.L. (1953). Intercalated discs in heart muscle studied with the electron microscope. *Anatomical Record*, **117**, 49–63.

Van der Stricht, O. (1895). La première apparition de la cavité coelomique dans l'aire embryonnaire du lapin. *Compte rendu de la Société de Biologie Sér. 10*, **12**, 207–11.

Van der Vusse, G.J. & Reneman, R.S. (1983). Glycogen and lipids. *Cardiac Metabolism*, chapter 10 (ed. A.J. Drake-Holland & M.I.M. Noble), pp. 215–37. Chichester: John Wiley & Sons.

Vassalle, M. (1976). Cardiac automaticity. In *Cardiac Physiology for the Clinician* (ed. M. Vassalle), pp. 27–59. New York: Academic Press.

Veress, A.T. & Sonnenberg, H. (1984). Right atrial appendectomy reduces the renal response to acute hypervolaemia. *American Journal of Physiology*, **247**, R610–R613.

Virágh, S. & Challice, C.E. (1973*a*). Origin and differentiation of cardiac muscle cells in the mouse. *Journal of Ultrastructure Research*, **41**, 1–24.

Virágh, S. & Challice, C.E. (1973*b*). The impulse generation and conduction system of the heart. In *Ultrastructure of the Mammalian Heart* (ed. C.E. Challice & S. Virágh), pp. 43–89. New York: Academic Press.

Virágh, S. & Porte, A. (1961*a*). Elements nerveux intracardiaques et innervation du myocarde. Étude au microscope électronique dans la coeur de rat. *Zeitschrift für Zellforschung und mikroskopische Anatomie*, **55**, 282–96.

Virágh, S. & Porte, A. (1961*b*). Structure fine du tissu vecteur dans le coeur du rat. *Zeitschrift für Zellforschung und mikroskopische Anatomie*, **55**, 263–81.

Virágh, S. & Porte, A. (1973*a*). The fine structure of the conducting system of the monkey heart (*Macaca mulatta*). I. The sino-atrial node and the internodal connections. *Zeitschrift für Zellforschung und mikroskopische Anatomie*, **145**, 191–211.

Virágh, S. & Porte, A. (1973*b*). On the impulse conducting system of the monkey heart (*Macaca mulatta*). II. The atrioventricular node and bundle. *Zeitschrift für Zellforschung und mikroskopische Anatomie*, **145**, 363–88.

Walker, S.M., Schrodt, G.R. & Edge, B.M. (1971). The density attached to the inside surface of the apposed sarcoplasmic reticular membrane in the vertebrate cardiac and skeletal muscle fibres. *Journal of Anatomy*, **108**, 217–30.

Warner, A.E. & Lawrence, P.A. (1982). Permeability of gap junctions at the segmental border in insect epidermis. *Cell*, **28**, 243–52.

Watanabe, T., Murushige, H., Naito, T., Sassa, S., Takahashi, S., Asazuma, S. & Hashimoto, I. (1978). Myocardial energy metabolism and protection of heart muscle at low temperatures. In *Recent Advances in Studies on Cardiac Structure and Metabolism*, vol. 12 (ed. T. Kobayashi, Y. Ito & G. Rona), pp. 485–9. Baltimore: University Park Press.

Weidmann, S. (1969). Electrical coupling between myocardial cells. *Brain Research*, **31**, 275–81.

Weihe, E., Reinecke, M. & Forssman, W.G. (1984). Distribution of vasoactive intestine polypeptide-like immunoreactivity in the mammalian heart: interrelationship with neurotensin- and substance P-like immunoreactive nerves. *Cell and Tissue Research*, **236**, 527–40.

Wendt-Galitelli, M.F., Stöhr, P., Wolburg, H. & Schlote, W. (1980). Cryomicrotomy, electron probe microanalysis and STEM of myocardial tissue. *Scanning Electron Microscopy*, 1980 (II), 499–510.

Westfall, T.C. (1977). Local regulation of adrenergic transmission. *Physiological Reviews*, **57**, 659–728.

Wilkinson, J.M. (1980). Troponin C from rabbit slow and cardiac muscles is the product of a single gene. *European Journal of Biochemistry*, **103**, 179–88.

Williams, A. (1983). Mitochondria. In *Cardiac Metabolism* (ed. A.J. Drake-Holland & M.I.M. Noble), pp. 151–71. Chichester: John Wiley.

Williams, E.H. & De Haan, R.L. (1981). Electrical coupling among heart cells in the absence of ultrastructurally defined gap junctions. *Journal of Membrane Biology*, 60, 237–48.

Willison, J.H.M. & Rowe, A.J. (1980). Replica shadowing and freeze-etching techniques. In *Practical Methods in Electron Microscopy*, vol. 8 (ed. A. Glauert), pp. 245–82. North–Holland: Elsevier.

Winegrad, S. (1970). The intracellular site of calcium activation of contraction in frog skeletal muscle. *Journal of General Physiology*, 55, 77–88.

Yamauchi, A. (1973). Ultrastructure of the innervation of the mammalian heart. In *Ultrastructure of the Mammalian Heart* (ed. C.E. Challice & S. Virágh), pp. 127–78. New York: Academic Press.

Yamauchi, A., Yokota, R. & Fujimaki, Y. (1975). Reciprocal synapses between cholinergic axons and small granule-containing cells in the cardiac ganglion. *Anatomical Record*, 181, 195–210.

Yee, A.G. & Revel, J-P. (1978). Loss and reappearance of gap junctions in regenerating liver. *Journal of Cell Biology*, 78, 554–64.

Yoshida, T. (1932). Fusion of the cardiac anlagen in the duck. *Anat. Arbeiten aus der Medizinischen universität zu Okayama*, 3, 61–91.

Yoshinaga, S. (1921). A contribution to the early development of the heart in mammalia, with special reference to the guinea pig. *Anatomical Record*, 21, 239–308.

Zak, R. & Galhotra, S.S. (1983). Contractile and regulatory proteins. In *Cardiac Metabolism* (ed. A.J. Drake-Holland & M.I.M. Noble), pp. 339–64. Chichester: John Wiley.

Zimmerman, A.N. & Hülsman, W.C. (1966). Paradoxical influence of calcium ions on the permeability of the cell membranes of the isolated rat heart. *Nature*, 211, 646.

Zisfein, J.B., Matsueda, G.R., Fallon, J.T., Bloch, K.D., Seidman, C.E., Seidman, J.G., Homey, C.J. & Graham, R.M. (1986). Atrial natriuretic factor: assessment of its structure in atria and regulation of its biosynthesis with volume depletion. *Journal of Molecular and Cellular Cardiology*, 18, 917–29.

Zypen, E. van der (1974). On catecholamine-containing cells in the rat interatrial septum. Enzymatic–histochemical and electronmicroscopical study. *Cell and Tissue Research*, 151, 201–18.

Zypen, E. van der, Hasselhorst, G., Merz, R. & Fillinger, H. (1974). Histochemische und elektronmikroskopische Untersuchungen an den intramuralen Ganglien des Herzen bei Mensch und Ratte. *Acta anatomica*, 88, 161–87.

INDEX